Alain Robert Makaba Ngoyi

Eating isn't rocket science

Alain Robert Makaba Ngoyi

Eating isn't rocket science

Who eats what, who eats whom and why?

ScienciaScripts

Imprint
Any brand names and product names mentioned in this book are subject to trademark, brand or patent protection and are trademarks or registered trademarks of their respective holders. The use of brand names, product names, common names, trade names, product descriptions etc. even without a particular marking in this work is in no way to be construed to mean that such names may be regarded as unrestricted in respect of trademark and brand protection legislation and could thus be used by anyone.

Cover image: www.ingimage.com

This book is a translation from the original published under ISBN 978-620-6-71708-9.

Publisher:
Sciencia Scripts
is a trademark of
Dodo Books Indian Ocean Ltd. and OmniScriptum S.R.L publishing group

120 High Road, East Finchley, London, N2 9ED, United Kingdom
Str. Armeneasca 28/1, office 1, Chisinau MD-2012, Republic of Moldova, Europe
Printed at: see last page
ISBN: 978-620-7-92290-1

Table of contents

FOREWORD

The second element of the ecosystem comprises all the living beings - plants, animals and micro-organisms - that find conditions in the environment that enable them to live and reproduce. Together, these living beings form a community (a term used mainly in America) or a biocenosis (a term used mainly in France). A biocenosis is a more or less species-rich ensemble of interdependent organisms, manifesting itself through competition, trophic relationships (some eat others), symbiosis, etc. The three categories of organisms in a biocenosis are producers (chlorophyllous plants), consumers (herbivorous and carnivorous animals) and decomposers (fungi, bacteria and certain animals).

From ancient times to the present day, food has been recognized as an essential component of health. From the 19th century onwards, basic science and technological progress have led to remarkable advances in nutrition, agronomy, food processing, transport and marketing. Despite this, new problems are emerging, linked to social phenomena, the industrialization of food and uncertainties about the properties and health risks of many products intended for human consumption.

What we eat has a major impact not only on our health, but also on that of our planet. To qualify as sustainable and healthy, a diet must meet a number of nutritional, economic, environmental and social criteria. With these theoretical elements in mind, let's take a closer look at the most common diets: what are the advantages and limitations of each in terms of health, social acceptability, economics and the environment?

In fact, some populations have preserved their traditional eating habits to this day, with small modifications linked to their culture.

In this book, we'll start with a look at the ecosystem, focusing on the food chain (from production to decomposition), food geography and diet from the first primates to modern man, to help the reader understand the evolution of man in relation to his natural and original diet. We'll also look at digestive physiology and certain diets, to answer the question: who **eats what, who eats whom and why eat?**

This manual is intended for nutritionists, health workers and nutrition advisors, agricultural professionals, health educators and all those with an interest in nutrition and health. It also complements other previously published resources in the fields of food and nutrition.

ALAIN ROBERT MAK

INTRODUCTION

The living beings that inhabit an ecosystem form the biocenosis (the environment being the biotope). All living beings in an ecosystem interact with each other, either directly or indirectly. They are linked by food relationships, or food chains.

A living ecosystem is healthy when all the organisms and inert media that make it up are in equilibrium. Ecological equilibrium is the natural balance between living beings and their environment, particularly within a food chain. If the climate allows abundant plant growth, the first consumers (herbivores), well fed, can multiply, but their predators take advantage to devour more and multiply too. If, on the other hand, plants become scarcer in a region, herbivorous animals that find little food become less numerous, and their predators, less well-fed, diminish even further.

Despite the importance anthropologists attach to culture as a determinant of eating behaviour, it is certain that the consequences of food intake are fundamentally biological.

The living organism is made up of thousands of proteins, fats, carbohydrates and other molecules, and synthesizes most of these substances from a relatively small quantity of elements and molecules known as essential nutrients. There's no doubt that we need a supply of energy, as well as amino acids and certain essential lipids, minerals and vitamins, not to mention water. To all this, we must add certain substances which are not essential to our diet but which play a role in its assimilation, such as certain fibers required, in appropriate quantities, for intestinal functions. Likewise, it is important to avoid ingesting a certain number of substances: not only toxic substances, but also those which, in moderate quantities, can play an important role for the body, but which, in excess, can become dangerous over the long term. In short, the nutritional needs of the human species are both quantitative and qualitative, or in other words, "human appetite" is not just a hunger for food, but for certain types of food. In other words, the omnivorous human being has had to learn to obtain all the nutrients absolutely necessary for survival (vitamins, amino acids, proteins, etc.) from a vast array of foods.

Food is essential to life. Its main role is to nourish the body. That's how important it is to our health. Food choices depend on many factors: culture, social environment, income, food availability and personal taste, as well as our natural and original genetic make-up. Food is therefore a subject that touches on many aspects of life.

This document does not pretend to cover the whole planet. It does, however, offer a quick overview of **WHO EATS WHAT, WHO EATS WHO AND WHY?**

The aim of this book is to help medical professionals and all our readers understand the concept of the ecosystem, human dietary behavior in the face of historical evolution from the first primates to modern man, and the advantages and disadvantages of certain diets adopted by humans in order to make the right choice when it comes to nutrition.

CHAPTER 1: STRUCTURE AND FUNCTIONING OF ECOSYSTEMS

1.1. General

A. Definition

Association of a specific physico-chemical environment (biotope) with a living community (biocenosis) (1).

Ecosystem=biotope + biocenosis

A forest made up simultaneously of trees, herbaceous plants, animals and soil.

- **Ecosystem:** forest.
- **Biocenosis:** phytocenosis (trees, herbaceous plants) + zoocenosis (animals).
- **Biotope:** soil.

Notion that can be applied to variable-sized portions of the biosphere.

Micro-ecosystem (e.g. tree)

Meso-ecosystem (e.g. forest)

Macro-ecosystem (e.g. region)

■ **Continental (terrestrial) ecosystems:** forest ecosystems (forests); grassland ecosystems (meadows); agroecosystems (agricultural systems);

■ Continental water ecosystems: Ientic ecosystems (lakes, ponds); Iotic ecosystems (rivers);

Oceanic ecosystems: seas, oceans.

2.2. Main ecosystems

A. Forest ecosystem

■ Land with more than 10% tree cover and a surface area of more than 0.5 hectares (ha).

- Trees must be able to reach a minimum height of 5 m at maturity.

B. Agro-ecosystem

- Ecosystem modified by man to exploit part of the organic matter

it produces, generally for food purposes.

C. Meadow

- Plant formations composed of herbaceous plants belonging
mainly to the grass family (grasses, cereals).

D. Ocean ecosystem

- The world's ocean is the planet's largest ecosystem, both in terms
of surface area (over 71% of the earth's surface = 360 million km^)
and depth (3,800 m on average).

E. Ientique Ecosystem

- All slow-moving or cloudy fresh waters (ponds, lakes, ponds...),

F. Iotic Ecosystem

- All running continental waters (rivers, streams, etc.).

1.3. Ecosystem structure

Écosystème

=

Biocénose

Producteurs de matière organique Consommateurs de matière organique Décomposeur de matière organique (recyclage)

Biotope

Énergie Matière organique /Inorganique

A. *The biotope: the environment occupied by living beings*

The biotope is the living environment made up of external conditions: temperature, humidity, light, soil, relief, etc.

A biotope is the physical and chemical environment in which plants and animals live. This environment is the non-living, or abiotic, component of the ecosystem. It contains all the resources necessary for life.

Biotope varies according to ecosystem. In a pond, it consists of water and dissolved substances (oxygen, carbon dioxide and mineral salts). In a forest ecosystem, the biotope consists of the soil, which enables plants to take root and provides them with essential water and mineral salts, and the atmosphere, which supplies oxygen and carbon dioxide (1).

B. *Biocenosis: all living organisms in an environment*

The second element of the ecosystem comprises all the living beings - plants, animals and micro-organisms - that find conditions in the environment that enable them to live and reproduce. Together, these living beings form a community (a term used mainly in America) or a biocenosis (a term used mainly in France). A biocenosis is a more or less species-rich grouping of interdependent organisms, manifesting itself in competition, trophic relationships (some eat others), symbiosis, etc. The three categories of organisms in a biocenosis are producers (chlorophyllous plants), consumers (herbivorous and carnivorous animals) and decomposers (fungi, bacteria and certain animals).

C. Trophic (food) chains

A trophic chain or food chain is a succession of organisms, each of which depends on the previous one.

A living being's place in a trophic chain represents its trophic level. There are three trophic levels:

- the level of producers, or primary producers

-consumer level (consumer 1, consumer 2, consumer 3, etc.)

- the level of decomposers.

Trophic chain components

1.   1 Autotrophic producers (Primary producers)

Primary producers are chlorophyll plants. They use light energy to transform mineral matter (water, mineral ions, carbon dioxide) into organic matter: this is the process of photosynthesis. Primary producers are autotrophs. They are the basis of organic matter production.

■ They form the 1er **trophic level** of the ecosystem (primary producers).

■ Autotrophic photosynthetic plants (Phototrophs)

■ **Ex**: Green plants, phytoplankton, cyanobacteria.

■ Thanks to photosynthesis, they elaborate organic matter from strictly mineral matter supplied by the external abiotic environment.

1. 2. Heterotrophic consumers

Heterotrophic consumers feed on organic matter. They are therefore entirely dependent on producers, either directly in the case of phytophages (primary consumers), or indirectly in the case of zoophages (secondary or higher-order consumers). Consumers are heterotrophs.

- Living beings that feed on the complex organic matter they obtain from other living beings.
- They see themselves as secondary producers.
- Consumers occupy a different trophic level depending on their diet.

   Exi : Consumers of fresh material

   Ex? : Consumers of corpses

- **Primary consumers (Cl):** These are the phytophagous that eat the producers. They are generally animals, called

herbivores (herbivorous mammals, insects, crustaceans: shrimp), but also more rarely plant and animal parasites of green plants.

- **Secondary consumers(Cl):** Cl predators.

   carnivores feeding on herbivores (carnivorous mammals, birds of prey, insects, etc.).

- **Tertiary consumers (C3) :** Predators of C2. These are carnivores that feed on carnivores (insectivorous birds, birds of prey, insects, etc.).

- In most cases, consumers are omnivores and therefore belong to several trophic levels.

- C2s and C3s are either predators (supra-predators) that capture their prey, or animal parasites.

- **Scavengers** are species that feed on fresh or decomposed animal corpses (dead organic matter). They often complete the work of carnivores.

- **Example:** Jackal$_5$ Vulture,...

1. 3 Decomposers

Use dead organic matter (from dead producers and consumers), transforming it into mineral matter. This is known as mineralization. We can distinguish between detritivores (vultures, dung beetles, earthworms), which consume corpses and excrement, and transformers (bacteria, molds, fungi), which complete the decomposition of organic matter until it is mineralized. This enables the material to be recycled (1).

- Various organisms and microorganisms that attack cadavers and excreta and gradually decompose them, ensuring that the elements contained in organic matter gradually return to the mineral world.

- All individuals that feed on animal or plant detritus.

- Their action marks the Ire stage in the transformation of dead organic matter:

Fragmentation of debris into finer elements released in feces (by enzymatic hydrolysis during intestinal transit).

Necrophagous: Feed only on animal corpses.

Ex: Necrophore, insect often associated with the tips of other adult insects or fly maggots on bird or mammal corpses. **Saprophagous:** Refers to living beings that eat decomposing plant matter.

 E.g. woodlice.

- **Geophages:** Soil animals that play a vital role in humification. **For example,** earthworms "eat their way through the soil". In this way, they digest fragments of plant matter that have been buried or fallen on the soil.
- **Coprophages:** Organisms that eat excrement.

E.g.: Dung beetle.

- The first stage in the degradation of dead organic matter, carried out by detritivores, enables microscopic beings such as bacteria, fungi and protozoa to carry out the second stage of this transformation. These micro-organisms are responsible for mineralization itself.
- The cyclic nature of the chain is ensured by the decomposers.

a. Chain of predators (consumers)

-Start with a (living) plant.

-The number of individuals decreases from one trophic level to the next, but their size increases (1).

E.g.: (1OOO) Carrots + **(10)** Hares + **(7)** Wolves.

b. Parasite chain

-Large organisms to smaller but increasingly numerous organisms (Elton's rule is not verified).

- Distant species can evolve inside each other's bodies (host/parasite).

Ex.:(l) Fir(Producer)/ **(10)** Caterpillar (Herbivore)/

(40) Braconids (Parasites)/ **(80)** Chalcidiens (Hyperparasites).

c. Chain of detritus feeders (saprophytic)

The circulation of matter is predominantly detrital. It goes from dead organic matter to increasingly small (microscopic) and numerous organisms (Elton's rule is not verified).

Ex: (1) Cadaver (fox) + **(80)** Nematodes + **(250)** Bacteria.

The structure of biocenoses is usually illustrated using ecological pyramids.

■ Superimposition of horizontal rectangles of the same height, but of lengths proportional to the number of individuals, biomass or quantity of energy present in each trophic level.

■ This is known as a pyramid of numbers, biomasses and/or energies.

■ Representations in the form of ecological pyramids make it possible to evaluate the reduction in matter or energy available to each subsequent rung in the food chain. Each rectangle of the pyramid will have a surface area proportional to the number of individuals, the total mass of individuals in the same category, or the quantity of energy. Ecological pyramids can therefore be used to quantify exchanges between trophic levels, or to assess the size of the populations concerned (2).

There are three categories:

1. **The energy pyramid** represents the amount of energy collected at each level of the food chain. Not all the solar energy collected by plants is available to herbivores: photosynthesis yield is low, and part of the energy is used to meet the needs of the plant itself. The second level of the pyramid is therefore smaller than the first. The same applies to the third, where first-order zoophagous (carnivores) do not harvest all the energy acquired by herbivores, etc. (2)

2. **The pyramid of numbers** represents the number of individuals at each trophic level. In any ecosystem, this number decreases from the prey level to the predator level. Population evaluation provides an

indication of the state of the ecosystem and can, for example, explain phenomena such as extinction or, on the contrary, outbreaks.

3. The biomass pyramid provides an assessment of the mass of producers in relation to that of consumers. The former is always greater than the latter.

CHAPTER 2: DIET FROM THE FIRST PRIMATES TO MODERN MAN

2.1 General information

To what period of our history should we refer to find a food model to which we can return to improve our health? When did we eat naturally, and therefore physiologically correctly?

If we go back in history, from antiquity to the present day, we see that nutritional deficiencies and illnesses were frequent, mortality premature, and the basic foodstuff little varied, essentially cereals.

The history of our last 2 millennia in the West does not allow us to find a reference model. But was the pre-historic Neolithic way of life more in line with our nature? Many nutritionists and physicians consider the introduction of cultivated cereals and farmed meat to be the beginning of serious collective dietary errors, epidemics and diseases of civilization (3). Is it possible, then, to find a model of our original diet during the Paleolithic period that conforms in every respect to our physiology and nature? During this period of more than 2 million years, the highly varied climates in which the members of our lineage lived conditioned their eating habits, which were strongly linked to nature4, so the models are diverse (4).

According to Lorain Cordain (5), "the basis of optimal human nutrition lies in the evolutionary history of our species and the pressures that have shaped our genome, and nothing in nutrition makes sense except in the light of evolution... (6).

It's on the basis of this idea, which seems to me to be full of common sense, that I'm embarking on a search for "the optimal diet for man, forged by millions of years of evolution", in an attempt to understand what the human organic diet is, the one that suits our genes, which haven't changed much in millions of years.

Sources of our knowledge on the evolution of food

What we know about the diets of hominids (7) and Paleolithic hunter-gatherers comes either from **anthropological** observations (skeletons, teeth, etc.) or from **archaeological** analyses (environment, habitat, fauna, flora, pollens, etc.), the techniques of which enable us to estimate the chronological evolution of diets.

1. Traces left on fossilized teeth

Scanning electron microscopy reveals the striations in tooth enamel caused by the type of food chewed. Long, vertical striations indicate a meat-based diet. Horizontal striations indicate a diet richer in vegetable matter. Eating leaves leaves polishing marks on the incisors. Omnivorous humans have had oblique striae since the beginning of the *Homo* lineage.

The chemical composition of teeth and bones gives an indication of the types of food usually ingested (7).

3-Type of teeth: massive, millstone-shaped teeth suggest a diet of grasses and seeds, while smaller teeth with pronounced canines and incisors point more to an omnivorousı diet....

Knowledge of the environment (fauna, flora) and of *hominid know-how (hunting_weapons, tools)* means we know what food resources are available.

2.2. Studies on living primates and ethnology.
A. Before the Paleolithic: the geological time scale.

1.   Beginning of the Cenozoic Era: appearance of primates (65 million years)

A very important event marks the end of the Cretaceous and Mesozoic eras and the beginning of the Cenozoic era. This was the Cretaceous-Tertiary extinction, around 65.5 Ma ago. It was massive, affecting a wide variety of animal and plant species in a short period of time on the geological scale. Mammal and bird clades, however, experienced few extinctions. Shortly after the disappearance of the dinosaurs, the first primates appeared at the beginning of the Paleocene, around 65 million years ago. The oldest known fossil of an ancestor common to all primates dates back 58 million years.9 To get an idea of their appearance and diet, let's take a look at their direct descendants, who have evolved little.

Prosimian monkeys: the most primitive branch of primates. They are divided into 3 families: the Lemuriformes (including the lemurs of Madagascar), the Iorisiformes (galago, loris potto) and the Tarsiiformes (tarsier).

a.   Lemuriformes have retained the ancestral traits of the first primates. They arrived on the island of Madagascar around 60 million years ago and evolved in isolation, without competition from other primates, which enabled several families to retain their primitive ancestral traits: they are arboreal, often nocturnal (lepilemur, microcebe...) and insectivorous. But their comb-like dentition also enables them to scrape gum from trees to eat it, which provides them with soluble fibers. Makis, on the other hand, are more advanced, diurnal and feed mainly on fruit.

b. **Iorisiformes.** Galagos live in equatorial Africa, and are very small (between a mouse and a rabbit), very lively and nocturnal. They supplement their vegetable diet (fruits, flowers, leaves) with insects and even small birds and lizards, which they hunt! They are adept at jumping and pounce on their victims from afar.

c. Tarsiers living in Malaysia and the Philippines share the same diet.

Conclusion: The food of the least evolved primates is insects, which were certainly the first food eaten by our Miocene ancestors 60 million years ago. They remain a natural food for us, and are still eaten by modern humans in many tropical countries (grasshoppers, termites, larvae...).

The most advanced, like makis, eat fruit.

The study of fossil primates shows that, around 50 million years ago, their diet was extended to include fruit, the gathering of which required more intellectual skill than the capture of insects.

Some prosimians eat eggs and hunt small vertebrate prey. This has also been observed in the fossilized remains of Miocene primates. These foods have been part of our dietary heritage since the dawn of time.

1. Miocene (between 23 million and 5 million years ago)
In the hundred or so primate species of this period, fruit seems to have been an important part of the diet, but the appearance of their teeth already argues in favor of a combined plant and animal diet, as in the earliest mammals.

The common ancestor of the great apes, Australopithecus and Man (Protohominoid) is thought to have been around 15 million years ago BP.

The oldest fossil of the human lineage, ***Tournai*** *{Sahelanthropus tchadensis),* was recently discovered and is dated at around 7 million years. In fact, *we are unable to say whether Tournai is the common ancestor of both* apes and humans, or only of the human lineage.

In those days, our "ancestors" ate plants, tubers, roots, insects and possibly small animals.

It was at the end of the Upper Miocene that the human and chimpanzee lineages separated. All the branches of the human lineage that we will review in our food history have disappeared. We are the only living representatives of the homo branch, although there have been several over the last 6 million years.

In order to complement the information provided by archaeology on rare fossils of the human lineage, and to approach our origins in a different way, I will first present the branches that separated from our lineage several million years ago, but which still have living descendants.

Humans, chimpanzees, orangutans and gorillas are the four surviving members of the Hominidae family. They have five identical chromosomes inherited from their common ancestor. The genetic make-up of the 3 great ape species is very similar to our own. Orangutans and gorillas give us information about the common ancestors of hominids. Chimpanzees separated from us more recently give us a closer look at Tournai.

-Orangutans live in the mountainous rainforests of Borneo and northern Sumatra. A separate branch from the other hominids 15 million years ago, they evolved independently in Asia. They are therefore genetically more distant from us than gorillas and chimpanzees.

Their day is devoted to foraging, feeding on leaves, bark, fruit, young thumbs, a few insects, seeds, bird eggs and small vertebrates, which they sometimes hunt. Just like some present-day prosimians.

The existence of a common ancestor for humans, chimpanzees and gorillas is proven by the indisputable presence of 11 common chromosomes and 7 mutated chromosomes.

They live in tropical African forests and are vegetarians: leaves, stems, roots, fruit and a few insects (termites) make up the bulk of their meals.

They are not hunters, and their digestive systems have evolved to adapt to this plant-based diet: their intestines and stomachs have developed to ferment the leaves they eat, so they are quite different from ours.

This bacterial fermentation also provides them with proteins.

Mountain gorillas (up to 3,500 m altitude) spend over 6 hours a day feeding on the leaves of wild celery, bamboo, berries, nettles and thistles, which are abundant all year round and rich in protein.

- Chimpanzees

Chimpanzees and humans belong to the Hominidae subfamily, which includes :

1. the Panine tribe (= genus Pan, with 48 chromosomes): chimpanzees and bonobos,

2. Hominins (= genus Homo, with 46 chromosomes): the various

australopithecine and human species

These 2 branches separated around 6.3 million years ago (8), when the two pairs of chromosomes {2p, 2q} of the common hominid ancestor merged to form the *{2}* chromosome pair of the Homo genus, which has since been reduced to 46 chromosomes. The genus Pan, on the other hand, has retained the 48 chromosomes of its common ancestor.

However, significant interbreeding between at least one chimpanzee species on the one hand, australopithecine species and probably Homo habilis on the other, leading to gene exchanges between the two tribes, must have existed for perhaps four million years (9)! It would have stopped two million years ago, coinciding with the first migrations of Homo habilis out of the chimpanzees' natural range with climate change. Common chimpanzees and bonobos, anthropoids from equatorial Africa, are the closest living animals to us physically and genetically. The chimpanzee genome differs from that of humans by less than 1%. The study of their diet is therefore an avenue for research into the closest food source to the origins of our human species.

The diet of today's chimpanzees

It was long thought that chimpanzees were vegetarians, but we now know that they are omnivores. They eat leaves (over 200 different kinds), fruit (around 65% of their diet) and buds, and are less active after their morning meal.

Chimpanzees were the first animals to be observed making weapons. They are highly skilled hunters, responsible for the disappearance of 20% of the apes living around them. In Senegal, females make wooden spears which they use to stab galagos (small primates) who take refuge in empty tree trunks 19. Meat seems to be a pleasure for them, and during the dry season in Côte d'Ivoire, it is indispensable to them, but they consume a wide variety of foods (over 300). With some of them they practice self-medication (medication copied by tradi practitioners) (7).

What can we learn from studying the diet of great apes?

The closest living hominids to us are omnivores and hunters. Our common ancestors were therefore certainly already meat eaters, long before the separation from chimpanzees, over 6 million years ago. We can assume that the proportion of animal intake in Tournai's diet 7 million years ago was close to that of today's great apes (15 to 20% maximum).

Among the great apes, there is one vegetarian species: the gorillas, but their digestive system has evolved since their separation from our hominid lineage to adapt to this diet, which is not original to great primates. Orangutans - which separated from us long before gorillas - still eat in a chimpanzee-like fashion, and consume a few animals, so this digestive aptitude for meat has existed in our ancestors for at least 15 million years.

In nature, a vegetarian diet has its drawbacks: you can't just pick up anything that grows near you, you have to look for something to balance your diet, avoid ingesting too much indigestible fibre, and pay attention to vitamin and mineral balance. That's why, for millions of years, the oldest primates in our line and the great apes have supplemented their diet with insects (abundant in tropical climates) and, for the most part, also with other animal foods...

Several developments have improved primate digestion, such as the modification of enzyme secretions and the incorporation of symbiotic bacteria to aid digestion. Humans have the same ability as apes to digest fibers, their commensal bacteria being able to ferment the fibers of 75% of plant membrane constituents, enabling 90% of fatty acids to pass into the bloodstream.

As with chimpanzees, in humans the speed of intestinal transit increases with the amount of fiber ingested. Thus, any reduction in food quality increases transit, and hence the digestive tract's capacity to ingest a greater quantity of matter.

Natural selection always favors traits that increase feeding efficiency. Primates have larger brains than other mammals, they develop greater cognitive abilities to solve their food problems and brain size is amplified by a diet that selects the best foods. This may have favored their adaptation to the changing climate in Africa, with the disappearance of the forest east of the rift. The emergence of the human species could thus be the result of the selection of individuals who had acquired a regular supply of foods of high nutritional value.

To finish with the great apes, I'd like to point out that the generally accepted pattern of human evolution, starting with an ape that gradually straightens out to become the modern bipedal sapiens, has been convincingly challenged by CNRS researcher Yvette Deloison in *"Préhistoire du piéton essai sur les nouvelles origines de l'homme"* (7). In it, she develops an original theory, solidly backed up by anatomy, physiology, embryology and genetics, showing that man has not acquired bipedal walking, but has on the contrary retained it since the earliest common ancestor of hominids (around 15 million years ago)(7), who lived on the ground, unlike apes, which have evolved tree-like movement and other adaptations to the three-dimensional environment of life in tropical forests (prehensile tails...). Evolution only goes in one direction - there's no going back once specialization has taken place (7). Our undifferentiated hand cannot therefore be the fruit of evolution, but rather of non-evolution, whereas in apes, the hand has become highly specialized in grasping branches, sometimes with the disappearance of the thumb. The fact that the common ancestor was bipedal may explain why the hand remained primitive and therefore unspecialized: it was never used as a foot, nor as a means of locomotion in trees (7).

Yvette Deloison shows that, among mammals (7), Primates have the most primitive foot bone structure, and that *"among Primates, it's Man who displays the maximum number of primitive characteristics, vestiges of adaptation to a distant aquatic life, which can be seen in the construction of organs such as the spleen, the kidney and the digestive tract. (This last point would be interesting to explore further, even if it goes beyond the scope of this thesis).*

   2. Pliocene (between 5.3 and 2.5 million years BP)

Hominids of this period still have a predominantly vegetarian diet, but some species seem to be eating more and more meat. Meat from herbivores was first introduced by scavenging (the simplest solution), then gradually by hunting.

Australopithecines are hominids closely related (biologically) to the genus Homo, but which have differentiated themselves from it by giving rise to a collateral branch.

-Australopithecines from the Afar region, such as *Lucy* **(3.2 million years BP (7)),** had very powerful jaws and large molars which they used to grind plant foods (nuts, tubers, roots); they consumed abundantly the underground parts of plants (roots, bulbs, tubers, rhizomes...) as well as other tough foods such as vegetables, and their strong incisors were perfect for peeling and cutting fruit. Leaves, fruit and roots are abundant in the tropics, but not very nutritious: you need to eat a lot of them to get the energy you need.

Australopithecines had to spend their days foraging for food and eating continuously while gathering.

B. Late Pliocene: The Lower Paleolithic

First period of prehistory, beginning **between 3 and 2.5 million years** before the present with the appearance of Man in Africa = **the genus Homo.**

Man's precursors are facing major climate change and aridification.

1. Homo habilis (2.4 to 1.6 million years BP)

A hominid from East Africa, Homo habilis evolved in a drier, less wooded savannah (rather than in the rainforest), unlike its ancestors. He was the first to have a cranial capacity of over 600 cm^3 . He was around 1.15 to 1.30 m tall and weighed 30/40 kg. He mastered stone-cutting, which could even be quite organized, and showed a certain technical skill as early as 2.3 million years BP. He had his own habits: the same sites were occupied for 10 to 15 years by the same groups, who hid tools and used them as larders. Homo habilis was not a nomad, but he did travel long distances to find the ideal stones for his tools.

Diet: Its masticatory apparatus reflects an increasingly omnivorous diet.

More than two-thirds of its diet is still made up of plants such as buds, young leaves, fruit and berries (in the wet season), and nuts, rhizomes and bulbs (in the dry season). However, the carbohydrate content of these plants is quite low, requiring a substantial intake of around one and a half kilos of plant matter per day.

Meat was an important part of their diet (probably around 400 g per day), and must have contributed to their survival and development. They probably primarily butchered the carcasses of large herbivores killed by the large carnivores (such as leopards) that were developing at the time. Unlike other predators, Homo habilis was able to access marrow and brains, and cut out tongues, thanks to its use of the flintknife. In experimental archaeology, it has been calculated that an impala butchered by hyenas could still supply 1,500 calories to a human who could break the bones to access the marrow and brain. Numerous animal bone remains have been found in Homo habilis deposits. The high consumption of bone marrow evidenced by the bones broken for this purpose may have played a role in the evolution of brain size. This intake of polyunsaturated fats (omega 3 and 6) was beneficial to the nervous system. They probably didn't just eat carcasses, but also hunted small animals.

2. Homo ergaster and Homo Georgicus (1.8 to 1 million years BP)

A new hominid species from East Africa, descended from Homo habilis.

A direct ancestor of present-day man. Perhaps the precursor of Homo Erectus.

Two skulls found in the Caucasus in 2000 have been dated at 1.7 million years, and this European branch has been named Homo Georgian. Until then, it was believed that our first ancestor to leave Africa was Homo erectus, 700,000 years ago, thanks to the appearance of Acheulean tools.

But this discovery shows that Homo ergaster preceded him by a million years, despite having much more primitive lithic instruments.

He was the first hominid to have a silhouette similar to that of modern man.

All the specimens found are large (1.70m), and their lower limbs indicate that they were excellent walkers, capable of running long distances.

Its cranial capacity of around 850 cm3 is smaller than that of Homo sapiens, but larger than that of its paranthropic contemporaries. Its skull also has features similar to those of Homo sapiens: a rounded frontal bone and a gracile jaw. Some believe that this species was the first to regularly consume meat. This may explain its survival and that of other hominids living in high latitudes, especially in winter.

Homo Georgian remains have been found in association with animal bones, stone tools and percussion implements that enabled this species to hunt, kill and prepare animals. This establishes Homo Georgensis as a hunter rather than a scavenger or a simple gatherer and consumer of low-grade plant foods. This explains why some individuals left Africa to follow herds of more appetizing herbivores than those of the savannah.

It would therefore have been the attraction of our very distant ancestors for game meat that drove them to leave their tropical territory 1.7

million years ago to face harsher climates...

3. *Homo erectus* (1.9 million years to 300,000 years BP)

They were the first hominids with skulls larger than 1000 cm3 (compared with our current 1350 cm3). They set up camp, built huts or occupied cave entrances. They were active gatherers and hunters, even of large game, thanks to the development of more sophisticated stone tools and weapons34. They also used natural traps (gorges or promontories) to hunt large herbivores: traces have been found of elephants, hippos and rhinoceroses being driven away from transhumance towards precipices or swampy terrain, where they could be finished off.

Food cooking as an evolutionary factor?

Homo erectus mastered fire and cooked certain foods. According to a recent hypothesis, cooking favored encephalization by making plant nutrients more available (particularly plant carotenoids). By cooking vegetables and roots, our ancestors would have given the brain easier access to important molecules for its development. Cooking makes starches more assimilable, certain plants more digestible and meats more tender.

What's more, cooked foods require less chewing effort and are easier to assimilate, so they deliver more calories more quickly. By reducing the time devoted to eating, cooking enabled people to devote more time to other activities, such as socializing, crafting or hunting. The invention of cooking thus played an important role in the evolution of modern man, freeing him in part from a major preoccupation: filling his stomach sufficiently. Chimpanzees spend almost half their time eating

(48%), whereas Homo erectus, like today's man, must have devoted less than 5% of its time to this task. Meals were therefore delivered more quickly, thanks to a major change in food preparation.

Anatomical clues can be found in the variation in molar size: in early Homo (H.habilis and H.rudolfensis). The gradual decrease in molar size is consistent with and can be explained by the evolution of the skull, but a sharp decline is observed in Homo erectus. The decline then continues irregularly in Homo sapiens. Nothing in phylogeny or the evolution of body size can explain such a change other than modified feeding behaviour. Food processing before consumption would therefore have become widespread from around 1.9 million years before present, at the time of the appearance of Homo erectus.

Fire makes certain indigestible or toxic foods edible (although some nutrients may be destroyed if cooked over a flame). Archaeology shows that different cooking techniques existed: pierrade, spit-roasting, stewing under ashes, boiling water in a wineskin with burning pebbles... Fire was also a place of socialization for the clan, and could foster communication and language... But the discovery of fire didn't stop mankind from still eating a lot of raw food.

Diet

Homo erectus continued to eat a lot of plants and fruit to provide the necessary plant fiber and vitamins (hominids of this period consumed 3 to 10 times more vitamins than we do), but he was also eating more and more meat. Dr. Delluc estimates that his diet was made up of around 35% animal products and 65% plant products, representing 700 g of meat and 1300 g of plants per day, corresponding to a normal carbohydrate intake of 50% of the calories in the diet.

If the percentage of meat increases, as is the case in colder climates than Africa, the body will have to resort to gluconeogenesis to obtain its carbohydrates.

The lakeshore and seashore also offered food that was easy to catch (periwinkles, oysters, cockles, crabs, seaweed...) and very rich in nutrients, including omega-3 fatty acids. Many researchers believe that this intake of DHA, particularly by women and children, who were traditionally responsible for harvesting these foods and had to eat them as they were gathered, played a decisive role in the evolution of the human brain. A pregnant woman who consumes omega-3 fatty acids provides her baby with a good supply of fatty acids, which in turn benefits brain growth.

Migration

Homos erectus migrated out of Africa, probably in small hunting groups following herds of herbivores northwards. The intensive practice of hunting led them to move over vast territories and modify their way of life. From this time onwards, the species hunted were highly varied, ranging in size from rabbits to mammoths. It was Homo erectus who gradually populated the Near East (7). In France, the best-known &*Homo erectus* fossil remains are those of the Tautavel man.

Sonship

The discovery of two fossils in 2007 on the eastern shore of Lake Turkana, Kenya, calls into question the relationship and order between the species of the genus Homo. Until then, it had been thought that *habilis,* then *erectus*, were first and foremost Homo (7).

Pathologies

A 500,000-year-old *&Homo erectus* skull found in Turkey shows lesions due to tuberculosis This is the oldest evidence of this disease in a hominid. *Homo erectus,* coming from tropical regions, probably had relatively dark skin, which was an advantage for sun protection in sunny countries, but a disadvantage for vitamin D production in colder countries.

As they progressed northwards, these migrants saw their vitamin D levels drop, and yet vitamin D is one of the first lines of defense against infections and certain diseases. This lack of vitamin D is certainly at the root of the first cases of tuberculosis.

Overall good health: they seem to have eaten well on the whole, with an energetic ration of around 3,000 calories covering the needs of these very active humans.

Between 400,000 BP and 250,000 years ago, the cranium expanded and the Iithic industry (Acheulean) developed.

C. *Middle Paleolithic: 300,000 to 28,000 years BP*

In Europe, it began with the widespread use of Levallois Iithic

debitage (48) and ended with the disappearance of Neanderthal man.

-Homo neanderthalensis

This extinct human being is distinct from present-day Man, whose ancestor he is not. Genetic analysis shows that he separated from the ancestors of *Homo sapiens* around 500,000 years ago. But his recently sequenced DNA shows no difference from our own...

He had a voluminous skull with a receding forehead (his cranial capacity of 1750 cm3 is greater than that of modern man), his supraorbital torus is very marked, and his chin practically absent. He was small with short, thick bones and a stocky silhouette, no doubt a force of nature that was highly resistant to the cold.

Neanderthal man is at the origin of a rich material culture called **Mousterian**, as well as the first spiritual concerns in Europe (first burials around 100,000 BC, as at La Ferrassie).

It was contemporary with *&Homo Sapiens* in Europe. Its disappearance is still the subject of controversy, but it is possible that the arrival of *&Homo Sapiens* ultimately proved fatal.

1. Neanderthal diet

It is the most carnivorous of all hominids. Biogeochemical analyses of bone collagen from Neandertals and associated mammals at the sites they occupied show a diet close to that of the wolf, even in temperate periods. Their **meat diet** consisted mainly of large mammals, but also included small animals (Iagomorphs, birds, terrestrial molluscs) when conditions were suitable. They also ate seafood, as attested in Europe as early as 150,000 BC. There are several indications that they also fished and ate fish, seals, dolphins... They even dried their fish, as shown by the particular wear marks on the teeth of a 45,000-year-old Neanderthal from Catalonia.

They also ate **plants** when they could find them, particularly in temperate regions. In 2010, analyses of phytoliths trapped in the tartar plates of fossilized Neanderthal teeth revealed traces of fossilized plants ^ date palm, legumes, water lily rhizomes, grasses of the genus *Triticum* or *Hordeum,* indicating a diversified diet and hunter-gatherer behavior.

Some of the starch grains found show cooking processes, suggesting that Neanderthals, thanks to their mastery of fire, cooked these plants by boiling them, whereas it was previously thought that only meat was cooked (based on the analysis of animal bones found in many homes).

2. Pathologies

Arthritis is particularly widespread among older Neanderthals. It specifically affects joints such as the ankles and spinal column.

and hips, arms, knees, fingers and toes. All of this is closely linked to degenerative joint disease (osteoarthritis), which can range from normal degeneration linked to wear and tear, to painful and disabling restriction of movement and deformity. They also presented with Dental Pathologies: signs of hypoplasia more or less pronounced on 75% of the teeth (10). Dietary deficiencies were the main cause, leading to tooth loss.

The question of vitamin D, Skin color plays a role in vit D synthesis: in equatorial regions, it is slowed down in melanoderms (dark skin), and in high latitudes, it is facilitated in Ieucoderms (light skin). The *MC1R (melanocortin-1 receptor)* gene on chromosome 16, identified in Neanderthals[61] and in redheads with pale skin and freckles, should facilitate this cutaneous synthesis of vitamin D.

D. *Upper Paleolithic 35,000 to 10,000 years BP End of last Ice Age*

A period characterized by the arrival of modern man in Europe, the development of new techniques (blades, bone industry, propulsion, etc.) and prehistoric art.

1. *Homo sapiens* or **modern man**

The only surviving species of the human lineage, archaic *VHomo sapiens* **appeared around 200,000 years BP, and** is thought to have evolved into anatomically modern man only in Africa, according to both genetic and paleontological evidence.

a. the diet of early modern man

They are certainly **omnivores.** But the proportion of animal and vegetable matter in their diet varies according to latitude and climate.

For an adult living a hunter-gatherer lifestyle, outside extreme environmental conditions, the average daily ration is 35% meat and 65% fibre-rich, low-sugar plants. To provide the 3,000 daily calories supposedly required, this corresponds to around 700 g of meat and 1,500 g of plants per day, which provides **35% protein** (¾ animal and ¼ vegetable), **22% lipids** (40% animal and 60% vegetable) and **43% carbohydrates.**

Paleolithic *homo sapiens* consumed 2 to 3 times less saturated fat than we do, and their carbohydrate intake was not much lower than today's, consisting almost exclusively of complex carbohydrates.

In the lands inhabited by the first *sapiens,* the range of edible plants was very wide, much wider than the narrow choice of plants later cultivated by farmers, and they were richer in protids than those we eat.

Vegetables contain proteins of lesser quality for us than those from animals, as they are often quite low in certain essential amino acids (especially tryptophan, lysine and methionine), which is a "limiting factor" for their use by our bodies. However, the combination of several plants can partly compensate for this deficit, hence the importance of diversity. Even if the bioavailability of plant proteins is only 70%, compared with 96% for animal proteins, this protein contribution is not negligible, given the quantity of wild plants absorbed per day.

Some dried plants, such as legumes (vetch, peas, lentils) or almost analogous (beans, walnuts, hazelnuts), have a caloric value and protein content quantitatively similar to those of meat, making them very interesting for building up reserves.

Shell mounds dating back 125,000 years have been found in Eritrea, indicating that the diet of Africa's earliest *Homos Sapiens* included seafood obtained by gathering on the shore.

b. Scattering on the earth

Homo sapiens left Africa **less than 100,000 years ago**, gradually replacing earlier human populations such as Neanderthal man. A great traveler, he populated the whole earth, but this time not just by following herds.

Since the earliest migrations, our ancestors have mastered navigation on the high seas, as demonstrated by the very early settlement of Australia.

A study of the human genome has just revealed that Australia's current Aboriginal population is descended from groups that have been settled for over 60,000 years (perhaps even 75,000). They are the oldest known population to have settled in the same territory over such a long period of time, apart from African populations.

The first *homo sapiens* to migrate northwards from Africa also mastered deep-sea fishing techniques. Thousands of bones of pelagic fish (such as tuna) eaten by humans around 42,000 years ago have been discovered on islands along the north-south migration routes in East Timor.

c. The environment in Upper Palaeolithic Europe

Homo sapiens arrived in Europe around 40,000 years ago, at the height of the Wurm glaciation. In other words, during the second half of the last of the ice ages that reigned intermittently throughout the Quaternary. These episodes, linked to changes in the earth's orbit around the sun, were characterized by colder temperatures and less precipitation.

During the 25,000 years of the Upper Paleolithic, the climate deteriorated until a "glacial maximum" around 20,000 years BP, then slowly improved during the Tardiglacial to the current climate (=! the Holocene).

Between 35,000 and 10,000 years ago, Europe was occupied by a homogeneous, modern-type human population with a common culture. Their most famous representative is Cro-Magnon man. In the area north of the Pyrenees and Alps where Cro-Magnon lived, the **climate was very cold and dry.** The landscape was Nordic, made up of monotonous steppes and tundra, lacking in edible vegetation, open to all winds and devoid of trees. The only remaining trees were conifers on the mountainsides or in the valleys (Scots pine, birch...). But this desolate landscape suited certain animals that made do with its sparse vegetation: mammoths, woolly rhinoceroses, herds of hundreds of thousands of wild horses, bison and reindeer. Polar foxes, wolverines, wolves and bears fed on hares, birds and baby herbivores (7).

d. Cromagnon man(69)

According to the skull found at Cromagnon, this is a man of modern anatomy. He had a tall stature, with marked muscular insertions, indicative of great robustness linked to great physical activity and a high protein intake; his intellectual capacities were the same as ours; he wore sewn and decorated clothes, and showed aesthetic preoccupations: jewelry, movable art objects and ritual cave paintings (Iascaux, La Madeleine caves...), musical instruments.... He sculpted the oldest known human face (-25,000 years) and structured his dwellings with activity zones around fireplaces, sleeping areas and dumping grounds. They lived in clans of 30 to 40 people. The best-known Cro magnon sites are in the Dordogne.

Cro-Magnon diet

Their mode of subsistence_appears to have been essentially based on the organized hunting of large land mammals. They practiced a nomadic lifestyle similar to that of sub-actual hunter-gatherers, due to the rapid depletion of game around the habitat, seasonal animal migrations and the appearance of food in certain places or regions of their territory. But they also fish with harpoons, hooks and fish traps... The basic food sources of European *homo sapiens* are game and wild plants, with a proportion of around 50% for meat and 50% for plants (according to Dr. Delluc). But this proportion varies according to climate. With each cooling, the scarcity of plants forces man to increase his consumption of meat, but as soon as the climate permits, he starts eating fruit, oilseeds, root vegetables, etc. again. Studies of the Inuit show that in the most extreme climate, the proportion of animal intake in the food ration is around 80%. For Cromagnon, this would only have lasted a few months a year, as plants were abundantly consumed in spring and summer.

Plants

Wild plants were richer in protein than our cereals, but also in vitamins and minerals. They were eaten soon after harvesting, without processing, which should have provided around 600 mg of vitamin C per day. Calcium and potassium intake was high, and in the absence of salt, the sodium/potassium ratio was at least 30 times lower than today. The Magdalenians of Lascaux, 17,000 years ago, benefited from a milder climate, with more forest replacing the Würm steppe. They ate walnuts, hazelnuts, acorns, beech faine and redcurrants. The Magdalenians of Miesenhaim (Rhineland), 11040 years ago, left 6000 seeds and 8000 pollens behind them. *"The Magdalenian could add to his animal diet salad with chicory, willow and clematis shoots (which are still eaten in Russia), young burnet leaves...".*

The study of dental tartar reveals phytoliths (siliceous secretions produced by plants) as well as starch grains that tell us about the wide variety of species consumed: wild grasses, tubers, roots... right down to water lilies.

The glucose needed by the brain came largely from triglycerides, as plants were rare and fast sugars unknown. Fruits were mainly berries: almost all the large, very sweet European fruits we know today did not exist in the European Paleolithic. The fast-sugar content of these berries was lower than that of today's fruits, and they were only present for a short period of the year. The Cro-magnon had mainly slow sugars, which could often only be used after preparation. The carbohydrate-rich chestnut has been known since the Miocene, but could only be eaten during glacial interstadials, as it requires a temperate climate.

Animal proteins: Meat that has been hunted or fished is remarkable for its high **protein** content and low lipid content. Indeed, Paleolithic meat is not the same as it is today*: "Wild animals that feed on wild plants produce lean meat with a fat content of no more than 4%, instead of 25% today".* Wild animals have no fat except reindeer, musk ox, mammoth and seal. The lipids in game are 3 to 5 times richer in polyunsaturated fatty acids than those in livestock.

The Paleolithic were unaware of the two disadvantages of animal proteins for us: their association with high lipid levels in farmed animals, and their cost price (it takes 10 kg of plant proteins to manufacture 1 kg of animal proteins). They drew on their natural resources, but did not renew them, so they varied in time and space. It is estimated that Paleolithic man obtained 30% of his calories in the form of proteins (i.e. 2 times more than today's recommended intake).

The study of animal bones collected in archaeological digs shows Cro magnon's particular appetite for young game, reindeer and horse, and among the preferred cuts: thighs, shoulders and head (for brains and tongue).

The search for **lipids** was important during ice ages. The fracturing of herbivore long bones indicates the search for marrow, a source of fat. Females were hunted, presumably for their fatter meat. *"At certain periods, prehistoric people consumed pregnant females, for their placenta and foetus. Very young animals were slaughtered, again for their high fat content.* These fats achieve an almost ideal balance between the two families of essential fatty acids, Omega 3 and Omega 6. *"Prehistoric man found these two families in a physiological ratio of*

1:1, whereas today's ratio is 20:1 in favor of Omega 6.

Paleolithic diets were relatively low in fat: 22% of calories, or 8% less than the recommended intake. But this level probably fluctuated according to time (cold or warm) and geographical area. The fattest fish, such as salmon, were preferred, as can be seen at Magdalenian sites. Salmon and eggs are 4 times richer in fat than mammalian meat.

Paleolithic man consumed a low proportion of saturated fatty acids (two to three times less than modern man) and a high proportion of unsaturated fatty acids (plant and animal).

Paleolithic food rhythms *"There were probably two norms among hunter-gatherers. Firstly, there was a single meal at the end of the day, with the hunters bringing back the produce of their hunt and/or the Gatherers bringing back their food for the communal meal. If the camp had food, then everyone stayed put and tended to snack all day. Three meals were therefore not the norm, and intermittent fasting was common, especially among hunters.*

e. Pathologies

Cro-Magnon was tall (1.70-1.80 m), had good bones and appears healthy from what we can tell from studying skeletons. Signs of bone deficiency are virtually absent. High meat consumption does not seem to have adversely affected his health, and there is no trace of gout or osteoporosis on his bones. This bone integrity testifies to proper nutrition and not to a so-called precarious "subsistence".

Researchers are wondering how they found sufficient calcium intake in their diet. Perhaps they were gnawing on bone epiphyses?

Most of the female figures, particularly those from Gravetti, are more or less gynoid in obesity, with ptosis of the breasts (a sign of repeated breast-feeding) and a rounded abdomen (a sign of advanced pregnancy). Although these statuettes are very realistic, this must not have been a frequent occurrence among these nomads on the move... Perhaps these statuettes represent their feminine ideal.

Obstetrical mortality must have been high: the skeletons found are usually those of young women. Infant mortality was high, and prolonged suckling spaced out pregnancies: the Paleolithic mother was certainly not surrounded by a flock of children! In fact, demographics increased only very slowly.

Some men died young too, but the skeletons show no traces of cancer, tuberculosis, nutritional deficiency, severe trauma or war wounds. Not all pathologies are imprinted on skeletons.

An analysis by INED reveals that once past the infant mortality hurdle, a 15-year-old could count on an extra 40 years of life, as was still the case in 17th-century France.

2. Ethnology: modern humans have preserved the Paleolithic way of life

Meat as a percentage of the diet

Anne Cayot Trottmann(2012) in her study of some fifty peoples without agriculture or livestock who survived after 1950, analyzed their diet based on game and uncultivated plants.

Meat intake varies greatly, especially with climate: among the Hadza of Tanzania, meat accounts for 20% of the diet, as it does among the Bushmen of the Kalahari; among the Australian aborigines of Arnhem, fish accounts for 30% of the diet, while among the Inuit, meat and fish account for 90%.

Gathering is considered by ethnologists to be a feminine activity, as pregnant women and women with children do not shed blood. But this does not mean it is a vegetarian activity. In fact, it has been observed that in addition to plant products, small animals are also collected: worms, insects and larvae, gastropods, amphibians, small reptiles and mammals. Protein-rich insects and fatty larvae have been and are eaten in Africa, Asia and Latin America (warm regions where they are abundant). In Africa, large crickets have always been eaten in a variety of ways: fried, boiled and salted, oven-roasted and sun-dried, then roasted with salt and cumin ground into flour for cakes...! They are an excellent source of protein.

In warm climates

Bushmen in the semi-arid Kalahari bush, women gather leaves, berries, almonds and walnuts, resin, tubers and bulbs on a daily basis, accounting for 80% of their food intake. Plants containing proteins, lipids and carbohydrates grow all year round, and the products of the hunt are not eaten daily, but are part of a feast[42] .

Australia's aborigines once knew how to identify 300 plants whose fruits, roots or tubers they ate. Alongside hunting by men, gathering and gathering provided 70-80% of the family's food, and throughout the day women and children roamed the desolate country to supply the evening meal with fruits, nuts, berries, seeds, yams and small warm- or cold-blooded animals.

In cold climates

a. In 1950, **Inuit** consumed 2 to 3 kg of seal or walrus meat (a quarter of which was fat) per day. According to observers from 1835-1855, they ate twice as much: raw or cooked, dried or pheasant meat, liver and viscera, stomach contents and blood, fish, birds, and systematic marrow and fat ingestion. During the short summer, meals were supplemented by eggs, cranberry mussels, 9 types of root and 3 types of seaweed. They are the most carnivorous of all Homo Sapiens.

b. The Ainu

Aboriginal population living in northern Japan and far eastern Russia. The climate is Siberian in winter, but conducive to the development of exuberant vegetation in summer. Their diet is closer to that of prehistoric *homo sapiens* than to that of Arctic populations. Just before the last war, they were still salmon and sea-fish fishermen, and hunters of deer, bear and marine mammals. They gathered a rich flora: shoots and leaves, roots and bulbs, numerous berries including wild grapes, berries and nuts, and oak acorns, which play an important role in the local diet. Fresh or fermented birch sap...

After these few examples of people still living as they did in the Paleolithic, let's continue our exploration of ancient times.

E. Mesolithic (10,000 years ago)

Between -12,000 and -9,000 years ago, **global warming** brought the Ice Age to an end: sea levels rose by 100 m to reach today's coasts, steppes were replaced by thick forests, and large, cold-loving animals (mammoths, reindeer) unfit for life in the forest migrated north to make way for deer, roe deer, wild boar, hares, bears and aurochs.

Man adapted, hunting methods changed, and the bow became highly effective on the new game - animals no longer lived in herds, but in isolation; the hunter had to track them and keep watch, and this mode of hunting required great skill and patience, and was no longer done in groups. *"This was a time of* diversity and abundance," explains Jean-Denis Vigne.

Rich vegetation grows on lake shores. Plants are more abundant and their consumption is increasing. The Azilian layer at Mas d'Azil in Ariège contained plum pits, sloes, cherries, walnuts, hazelnuts, acorns, and a very small pile of wheat...

From that time until recently, a wide range of plants have been gathered, including edible mushrooms, fruits and berries (apples, pears, cherries, sloes, medlars, comouilles, strawberries, raspberries, blackberries, blueberries, redcurrants, etc.).) herbaceous or woody plants whose leaves and flowers are picked: lungwort, watercress, raipon, nettle, violet, oxalis, primrose, young shoots of ash and fir... Aromatic plants: juniper, marjoram, wild mint, wild garlic, chives, woodruff, etc.

They also eat seeds and dried fruits such as chestnuts, faines and hazelnuts. They also eat acorns, which are dried and ground into flour to make bread or cakes when cereals are not available. And roots, bulbs and tubers such as walnuts, raipberries, genets, dog's teeth and even fern rhizomes (which were ground to make bread in times of famine in the 18th century).

Analysis of fossil fecal matter from this period shows that humans ate raw. Cooking was not at all systematic, even after the invention of fire. Demographics were on the rise, thanks in particular to a subsistence mode that relied heavily on the exploitation of plants. The number of occupied sites was significantly higher than in the Paleolithic. Receding glaciers enabled people to migrate further north. Instead of being satisfied with this warming, humans moved to occupy the whole of Northern Europe and the mountains freed from their glaciers!

F. The Neolithic (in France between 5500 and 1800 BC)

hen, less than 10,000 years ago, people gradually began to settle down and domesticate plants and animals, a change that began in the Fertile Crescent. This new way of life then arrived in Europe in small groups of farmer-breeders from Anatolia and south-west Asia. Its spread across Europe, from the Aegean Sea to the British Isles, took around 2,500 years (between 6,500 BC and 4,000 BC). More than a "Neolithic revolution", it was a slow, geographically disparate evolution that took hold throughout the world.

1. Food: agriculture and livestock

The change in lifestyle was accompanied by profound changes in human diet, with the production of mealy cereals (slow carbohydrates) and fatty animals, and the possibility of building up reserves. Meat consumption dropped drastically, and plants (mainly cereals) accounted for up to 90% of the diet. The increase in horizontal dental striae and decrease in vertical striae reflect the decline of hunting in favor of agriculture.

But this evolution towards a "typical" Neolithic regime occurs slowly. The Pendimoun site (Alpes-Maritimes, France), for example, shows an infinite number of transitional situations with the Mesolithic: "At the start of the Early Neolithic, we see the beginning of the domestication of Ovicaprinae and cattle, but also a lot of **wild fauna,** pigs, deer, roe deer, rabbits, hares, large ruminants, a few cats, foxes and marten for fur. There are also remnants of cereal crops (einkorn, starch wheat, barley). On the other hand, studies show that very little use is made of marine resources, even though we're close to the sea. This is the beginning of a specialization".

This new peasant way of life, which took hold during the Neolithic period, remained unchanged during the Metal Age and until the end of the 19th century.

a.Plant domestication began with starch wheat, small spelt and barley. They were chosen not primarily for their nutritional quality, but because they had larger seeds and were easier to handle. Strains that retained their edible seeds longer were selected.

Then came the leguminous plants: peas, lentils and beans,_which had the advantage of being eaten fresh or dried and could be stored. Rye, for example, was tried and abandoned in Neolithic Anatolia, but made its way to Europe as a weed and was successfully domesticated there, thousands of years after the birth of agriculture. Wild lentils took just as long to domesticate.

b. In the Paleolithic era, consumable **vegetation** (fruit, leafy shoots, roots, etc.) consisted almost exclusively of dicotyledons, and primates had had plenty of time to get used to them for tens of millions of years. In the Neolithic era, the massive use of monocotyledons (cereals), which are not easily digestible by humans (who are not granivores), made it necessary to use mortars and pestles, which did not exist before, to obtain flours.

c. The invention of ceramics: utilitarian pottery became widespread around 6000 BC. The storage of harvested cereals in ceramic vessels replaces the pit dug in the ground. It was safer from animals and bad weather.

The seeds were roasted for better preservation.

Cooking food is made easier by the use of fire-resistant containers. Even liquid foods could be cooked for longer without carbonizing. A "new cuisine" emerged, with purées and porridges. Cereals contain less fiber than wild plants and are higher in calories, so we eat less of them to satisfy our hunger, and fiber intake declines.

The consumption of vegetable porridges is attested by **mummified Neolithic corpses** found perfectly preserved in the peat bogs of northern Europe. The contents of their internal organs, including their stomachs, have been studied.

The man from Tolund (Denmark, died around 350 BC) was of high status, as shown by his hands, which are not those of a manual laborer, yet his last meal consisted of barley, linseed, knotweed and numerous weed species (umbelliferae, daisy, bindweed, patience...).

The man from Graubelle had eaten 66 different types of seed porridge (buttercup, ryegrass, chamomile, etc.) and the Woman from Boron a similar seed porridge. Most of the seeds were tiny, some rich in oil.

This shows that agriculture has by no means eliminated the need to gather wild plants.

d. Breeding

The first domesticated species are goats, sheep, pigs and cattle... all of which were domesticated at roughly the same time, around 8500 BC, in the Near East. These were the animals that existed naturally in the region and were the easiest to approach. The meat was probably smoked to preserve it. Salt was not used as a preservative until around 2000 BC. But animals are expensive to feed, so hunting and fishing continue.

e. Milk began to be consumed 7500 years ago in central Europe, as a logical consequence of cattle breeding. Until then, the only humans to consume milk were breast-fed infants. We don't know how much milk was consumed in the Neolithic period, but not all adults today have the enzymes (Iactase) to digest this non-physiological food. A few thousand years is not enough to change our digestion.

f. Population growth

The work of paleodemographer Jean-Pierre Bocquet-Appel indicates a probable correlation between the beginning of agriculture and the demographic surge of populations. There was a sharp increase in fertility, thanks to shorter birth intervals. Recovery from childbirth (relevadles) is more rapid, which can be explained by more regular feeding due to greater food storage capacity.

2. Pathologies

The "agricultural revolution", which led to a predominance of cereals in the diet (50-70% of food intake), was accompanied by a deterioration in health, as evidenced by skeletons: for the first time in human history, traces of **iron-deficiency anemia, rickets** (due to wheat lectins, which block vitamin D), **chronic inflammation** (too much omega 6) **and osteoporosis** (calcium and vitamin D deficiency) appeared.

a. Human **stature** decreases by a good fifteen centimetres from this period onwards, partly due to low protein intake, but also undoubtedly due to the transformation of physical activity: the stamina of sedentary farmers replaces the endurance of semi-nomadic hunter-gatherers.

Agricultural work creates new stresses, with children undoubtedly starting to work early and being subjected to physical portages that block growth.

-**Tooth decay,** which was very rare in the Palaeolithic period, multiplied in the Neolithic. **Teeth and bones** also bear the marks of deficiencies caused by refining and phytic acid in cereals. **Phytic acid** is an anti-nutritional compound that traps minerals. Cereal grains contain 1 to 5% phytic acid, which is used to store phosphorus. Mammals (including humans) cannot hydrolyze phytic complexes (except ruminants, which have the necessary microbial flora). Phytates are capable of causing deficiencies in calcium, iron and zinc, despite correct intake. This may have played a role in the increasing reduction in human height since the Mesolithic period, as well as in the drop in animal protein intake, food shortages linked to climatic hazards and epizootics, and exposure to epidemics due to proximity to animals.

Sedentarization leads to contamination by human and animal faecal germs. This was the beginning of **infectious diseases,** linked to promiscuity with animals in villages, population mixing and increased population density. Tuberculosis, for example, which was absent in the Palaeolithic, is undoubtedly of animal origin, as are many infectious diseases (smallpox, leprosy, salmonellosis, tapeworms, typhoid, anthrax, influenza, rabies, tetanus, syphilis...) domestication may not have been such a good thing for our health...

Among the **new diseases** visible on the skeletons: hemolytic anemias, ankylosing spondylitis, Fiessinger-Leroy-Reiter syndrome...

Grinding grain on the knees, all day long, causes osteoarticular lesions in women's toes, spine and knee. Farmers suffer from lumbosacral arthrosis due to the constricting positions in which they work. This was the beginning of occupational diseases.

We find **polypathologies:** as in the case of Ôtzi, a forty-year-old man, 5,300 years old, found mummified in a glacier in the Alps, murdered by a flint arrow in the back (near the axillary artery). Diffuse osteoarthritis, atherosclerosis, chronic bronchopulmonary disease, enthesopathy (inflammatory disease) in the knees, presence of three gallstones indicating that Ôtzi's diet was rich in protein, intestinal parasites.

Electron microscopic examination of the hair revealed a neurotic pathology, and examination of the nail an abnormality characteristic of intense stress 8, 12 and 16 weeks before his death. This poor general condition seems to be linked to the presence in his intestine of trichinella eggs, a parasite that produces attacks every twenty days.

Otzi is also the first man known to have been infected with the Lyme disease parasite. He also has a series of recalcified rib fractures on his left side.

An hour before his death, Otzi had eaten a meal consisting mainly of wild goat. His viscera contained vegetable matter (75% of which was cereal), deer and ibex.

In conclusion: His state of health was as bad as that of our contemporaries, if not worse, despite a life in the fresh mountain air and meat that was still wild. This did not prevent him from leading an active and warlike life.

The Neolithic was also a time of **food shortages, deficiencies** and

epidemics, as evidenced by collective burials, **flints stuck in bones** and mass graves. The Neolithic period also saw the first **wars.** The building up of reserves and therefore wealth was unfortunately at the root of the first conflicts.

Even after sedentarization and the invention of agriculture, the gathering of wild plants continued for a long time, as shown by the men of the peat bogs, and still exists in our countryside (dandelions, nettles, watercress...) and in many countries today, as in Crete for example. The diversity of plants consumed is very important for human health. Agriculture has brought food security and abundance, a source of demographic growth, but we mustn't be satisfied with a choice of foods, as Neolithic man knew. The current depletion of plant resources is not in line with our needs. 5 major cereals provide most of the world's food today.

Unleavened cereals (such as porridge) cause mineral deficiencies, as humans are not at all prepared to digest them properly. We've only been eating cereals for 7,000 years, which isn't long enough for our physiology to have adapted.

Animal husbandry was not intensive in the Neolithic, as the high cost of producing meat for animals to be fed restricted consumption, and hunting continued to be practiced. But living in close proximity to animals was a vector for previously unknown diseases.

The use of animal by-products such as milk spread gradually, but certainly not to the same extent as today. Under natural conditions, animals produce little milk, and only for a few months of the year.

The health picture of the Neolithic period looks bleak, as the proponents of Paleolithic food point out. But there are those who defend this period and do not believe in the harmful effects of foods derived from agriculture and animal husbandry.

After the introduction of new foods such as cereals and milk, which upset our original eating habits, the next major changes in diet came in the 20th century, when industrial expansion brought with it a surfeit of even less physiological foodstuffs.

G. *The industrial revolution*

In the 19th century, with the industrialization of production, including food, man once again rapidly modified his diet. The foods we eat are impoverished and denatured by all kinds of treatments and modifications. Our digestive enzymes no longer recognize them, our organs are attacked, and our blood, poisoned and thickened, circulates poorly.

1. The destruction of our food by the agri-food industries

a. **Intensive farming** denatures food with fertilizers, fungicides, pesticides, hormones and chemicals of all kinds, leaving it deficient and toxic,

b. Long-term **food preservation** by freezing, freeze-drying, appertizing, irradiation and the addition of chemical preservatives affects the nutritional quality of food,

c. **Refining** eliminates enzymes, vitamins and minerals, producing purified products devoid of nutrients (white sugar, white flour, purified oils, pasteurized cheeses, etc.).

d. **Systematic cooking** destroys nutrients: destructuring of proteins, lipids and carbohydrates, with the formation of tars (proteins) and the Maillard reaction.

2. New eating habits

a. Salt

Man has been exploiting salt deposits since the end of the Bronze Age, but it remained a rare and expensive product, so was consumed sparingly until the industrial age, when its consumption exploded, to the detriment of our health.

The balance of the internal environment, in particular hydration through sodium metabolism, is governed by the kidney. The sodium filtered by the glomerulus is almost entirely reabsorbed by the proximal tubule and the loop of Henlé, while the distal tubule merely adjusts according to need (via the renin-angiotensin system). The workload of the renal tubule is considerable: of the 1,000 g of salt filtered per day, our kidneys eliminate only a few grams in the final urine. So, like the kidneys of animals in hot climates, our kidneys are designed for a low daily intake of salt, and operate on an economy basis. To compensate for daily losses, 1 to 1.5 g of sodium chloride per day are sufficient. Sodium chloride is provided by the natural diet, without the need for supplements. Wild plants provide approx. 10 mg sodium per 100 g, and (domestic) animals 69 mg per 100 g.

In the Paleolithic era, a diet consisting of 35% meat products (approx. 788 g) and 65% vegetable products (1463 g) would have provided a total of 690 mg sodium per day, or 1.7 g sodium chloride. This was sufficient.

Today, however, we consume between 10 and 45g a day. This leads to high blood pressure and cardiovascular complications.

b. Fast sugars have been absent from the diet since our origins, except for honey, which has been consumed since ancient times, but has always remained a rare product.

Cane and beet sugars spread with the industrial revolution, their consumption is constantly increasing and their impact on health is enormous.

In less than 200 years, we've moved further and further away from fresh, natural products.

Our bodies cannot adapt to the radical industrial transformations of modern food. Our food is polluted, refined, over-sweetened, over-salted, enriched with poor-quality fats, preservatives and colorants... destroyed by increasingly aggressive cooking methods such as the microwave...

There's not enough time to cook for yourself, and ready-made industrial products have replaced traditional foods such as fruit, vegetables, pulses and wholegrain cereals. Our diet lacks vegetable fiber. Fats rich in saturated and trans fats have replaced unrefined oils (rich in omega 3, 6, 9). Plants come from all over the world, and the abundance of food in all seasons has made us forget the rhythm of nature... In 3 generations, our ancestral culinary references have been lost; our diet is fast and non-diversified, nibbling at all hours on toxic and non-digestible foods disrupts all our digestive organs...

The variety of industrial products is constantly increasing, while that of natural products is shrinking dangerously. Of the 70,000 edible plant species on earth, only 10% are cultivated. But just 30 species provide

95% of human energy needs. This hyperspecialization of the agri-food industry has led to the neglect of tens of thousands of plants whose variety and richness we need. Producers select species that adapt easily, keep for a long time and yield massively per hectare, with no concern for our nutrition. The profit motive produces seeds degenerated by genetic manipulation, vegetables with calibrated, insipid, rot-proof shapes... and traditional seeds are banned... The agri-food multinationals that orchestrate all this are the predominant components of the international economy, and they control the media and the organizations that draw up nutrition programs. The most profitable foods for these industries are those based on wheat, milk and sugar, and are therefore the most recommended and consumed...

They are also the least adapted to our physiology, and the most recently introduced in the history of our diet. But in our affluent societies, people no longer eat by instinct but by "impulse", bludgeoned by advertising and all kinds of contradictory nutritional messages.

Knowledge of our past is useful in helping us to step back from these new eating habits and return to more common sense and critical thinking in our food choices.

3. Pathologies

In the second half of the 20th century, we were force-fed cheap, unphysiological food, the visible effects of which on public health can no longer be disputed. After the appearance of tooth decay in the Neolithic era, it's now the so-called "diseases of civilization" that have made their entry in force over the last fifty years, and they're on the increase. Obesity and overweight, diabetes II, cardiovascular pathologies, inflammatory, digestive, autoimmune and neurodegenerative diseases, cancers, food allergies... Health is deteriorating fast, but as longevity increases with the progress of emergency medicine, the elderly are suffering from multiple disabling pathologies and long agonies.

We've been omnivores since our earliest origins, millions of years ago. Our digestive physiology enables us to digest and assimilate all types of natural foods, making us highly adaptable to environmental changes. But the ratio between animal and vegetable intake has slowly evolved over time towards an increasingly camel-like trend, and the earliest tools of our first *homo* ancestors were designed for butchering carcasses and crushing bones.

Early man was distinguished by his search for quality, nutrient-rich foods, which helped develop his brain. Low-carbohydrate, low-calorie plants were not enough for them. The consumption of bone marrow certainly contributed to brain growth, as did wild game rich in omega 3 and low in saturated fats, and shellfish and fish rich in omega 3.

Meat provides glucose through gluconeogenesis in times of drought and lack of vegetation, and helps maintain a regular food supply whatever the climate. The emergence of the human species could be the result of the selection of omnivorous individuals having acquired a regular supply of foodstuffs of high nutritional value.

With *homo georgiens* 1.7 million years ago, the hunting character of our ancestors is clearly apparent and their attraction for game is such that they leave Africa to venture into colder climates, abandoning the tropics and their luxuriant vegetation for good game fed on green grass... Its gracile jaw, like that of homo sapiens, shows that it already eats less tough vegetation, which it has replaced with meat.

With *homo erectus*, the consumption of herbivorous animals became even more important, with social organization based on the hunting of big game. Cooking food, particularly plants (including starches), also favored encephalization by releasing plant nutrients. As a result, more calories are absorbed more quickly, and man spends less time feeding and chewing; his dentition diminishes sharply from this point onwards. *Homo erectus* emigrated far from Africa, adapting to all climates thanks to an omnivorous diet with a strong cameloid tendency. A frugivorous vegan hominid would not have been able to survive in the north, and would not have felt the need to move far from the tropics.

Homo sapiens, i.e. modern man, is not the descendant of a branch of &homo erectus that emigrated north hundreds of thousands of years ago, but rather is extinct. *Homo sapiens* appeared in Africa from &homo left behind around 200,000 years ago, and stayed there until around 60,000 years ago, when some of them began to spread across the globe. Today's Africans are those who did not emigrate and have remained adapted to the lifestyle of our common ancestors. *Homo sapiens* arrived in Europe at the height of the Ice Age around 40,000 years ago. Despite this major environmental change, they adapted well. The Cro-Magnon hunter-gatherers of the Dordogne could consume more than a kilo of meat a day, but frequent periods of fasting linked to an uncertain supply and intense physical activity in the cold enabled them to burn off and autolyze the toxins generated by the digestive metabolism of meat. In fact, it seems that they never exceeded 50%

meat in their diet, despite their poor vegetation.

The research I did for this thesis answered one of my biggest questions: why did our ancestors, who I thought were vegetarians by nature, immigrate to Europe in the middle of the Ice Age? In fact, if they had been vegetarians, they wouldn't have gone north. There was no demographic pressure to push them out of Africa, only the lure of fatter herds in colder regions could attract them to this harsh climate. It was the abundant consumption of fresh meat that they enjoyed so much that enabled them to survive the Siberian winters. (It's a choice I personally regret, as I like neither cold nor meat...).

In conclusion, we who, during the Paleolithic period, i.e. for 99.5% of our human trajectory, were hard-earned consumers of game, fish and wild fibrous plants, are now, for the last 0.5% of our evolution, becoming sedentary people with changed habits and degraded health and vitality. Our nutrient requirements have not changed since the appearance of *Vhomo sapiens*, and probably very little since the first *homo* 2 million years ago. However, this is a characteristic of our. Genetic evolution is very slow Humans and chimpanzees split up 6 million years ago, and species diversified to adapt to a wide variety of conditions. We quickly made the transition from the Paleolithic to the very different Neolithic diet. Our meat consumption dropped sharply to meet the demands of a much larger population, and the basis of our diet became plant-based, while animals, which are expensive to feed, were reserved, as in today's traditional populations, for special occasions, chefs and the rich. So, while we were already experiencing major dietary changes 10,000 years ago, up until the last century we always ate natural, unpolluted foods. The dietary upheaval of the 20th century is certainly the most brutal and hardest on the human organism that we have ever experienced.

In short, the history of food can be divided into three ages of very unequal duration:

-the pre-agricultural age, between 3 million years BP and 10,000 years BP,

-the agricultural age between 10,000 BP and the 19th century, and the agro-industrial age for the last 150 years.

If we make a chronological comparison with a time scale reduced to one year :

CHAPTER 3:[t] PHYSIOLOGICAL AND NATURAL HUMAN NUTRITION

3.1. Physiology of digestion and mechanisms of intestinal absorption

A. *Introduction*

The proteins, carbohydrates and fats we ingest every day are broken down into nutrients in the digestive tract and absorbed by the small intestine. The nutrients thus absorbed are then distributed throughout the body via the bloodstream or lymphatic system.

B. *General information:*

1. **Digestive work:** Mechanical and chemical transformation of food for absorption.

   - Digestion: transformation of food (proteins, lipids, carbohydrates) into nutrients (amino acids, fatty acids and cholesterol, glucose).

   - mechanical: provided by the muscular fibers of the digestive tract.

   - chemical: ensured by the action of digestive enzymes.

   "Coordinated by SN and hormonal."

   - Absorption :

   Nutrients are captured by intestinal cells (enterocytes), then transferred to the internal environment (blood and lymph).

2. Diagram of the digestive system.

Mouth cavity → oesophagus → stomach → small intestine → large intestine consisting of ascending colon then crosses from right to left flank, then descending then sigmoid then rectum and finally anus. All along the tube are sphincters (= muscular reinforcement).

-Upper esophageal sphincter

-Lower esophageal sphincter = cardia

-Pylorus

-Ileocecal valve

-Anal sphincter.

It is a long muscular tube of variable diameter in three portions:

-ingestive (mouth + esophagus).

-digestive (stomach + small bowel + colon).

-ejective (sigmoid).

Three glands in the oral cavity:

-sublingual.

-under the maxilla.

-parotid.

Two glands external to the TD :

-Liver → bile + liver secretions.

-pancreas → pancreatic secretions.

Both discharge their secretions into the duodenum, jejunum or ileum via the sphincter of Oddi.

3. Wall :

Three layers:

-serous (outer layer surrounding the TD), secretes a small amount of liquid to lubricate the outer surface of the TD

-middle layer = muscularis: ensures the motor phenomena of the TD.

Between the two layers of this muscular layer are the nerve clusters that form Auerbach's plexus.

-inner layer = mucosa: contains blood vessels, lymphatics, glands and Meissner's plexus.

4. Glands.

Mucous membranes :

Stomach: fundic glands (in the fundus) and pyloric glands (terminal part of the stomach, the pylorus).

f Small intestine: Brünner's and Lieberkhhn's glands. Appendices:

Liver and pancreas, whose secretions are discharged into the duodenum.

C. Digestion :

From mouth to anus, food undergoes multiple chemical and mechanical transformations. These modifications can be divided into 3 phases, depending on where the food is transformed into nutrients:

- The mouth and esophagus phase

- The gastric phase

- The intestinal phase

1. **Oral and esophageal phase :**

Salivary secretions

Sight, smell, hearing (the sound of grilling meat) or simply conditioning trigger an influx that is integrated into the cerebral cortex, generating a vagal response. This response leads to an increase in salivary, gastric and pancreatic secretions, as well as contraction of the gall bladder and relaxation of the sphincter of Oddi.

The arrival of food in the oral cavity intensifies this phenomenon, as food comes into contact with the epithelium. This induces a local reflex increase in salivary secretions from the accessory salivary glands. The daily volume of saliva thus produced can reach 1500 ml of alkaline secretions (pH between 7 and 8).

Composition and role of saliva

Substances	Role
Mucine	Lubrication
Salivary amylase	Starch digestion
Lingual lipase	Lipid digestion
Lysozyme	Antibacterial

IgA	Antibacterial

> ## Mastication

- Mastication breaks down food into small particles.

- It helps form a food bolus for swallowing.

- Saliva begins the digestion of lipids and starch.

- It facilitates gustation by solubilizing particles.

- It cleanses the mouth and has an antibacterial action.

- Its alkaline pH neutralizes acid reflux into the esophagus.

- Ingesting food produces stimuli for gastric and duodenal functions.

> ## Swallowing

The pharyngeal stage of swallowing begins when the food bolus is voluntarily pressed against the roof of the mouth.

This causes a wave of involuntary contractions that block the access of food to both the upper and lower airways, pushing the food bolus into the esophagus.

The food bolus then descends to the stomach; to do this, the esophagus has 2 types of peristaltic movement: primary and secondary.

> ## Role of the esophagus

- propulsion of food into the stomach

- **Upper esophageal sphincter (SOS)** Protects the upper

respiratory tract by preventing food from entering.

- **Esophageal body:** thanks to secondary peristaltic waves, it prevents gastric reflux from ascending into the esophagus when the lower esophageal sphincter does not adequately fulfill its role as an anti-reflux barrier.

- **Lower esophageal sphincter (LES)** Acts as an anti-reflux barrier

2. The gastric phase of digestion :

➢ Role of the stomach

The stomach receives the alimentary bolus, which it mixes with its secretions and transforms into chyme. The stomach can be divided into 3 functional parts:

• **The cardia region** Located at the entrance to the stomach, this portion secretes mucus, which helps food slide into the stomach. In addition, the cardia prevents gastro-oesophageal reflux by its anatomy and its alkaline secretions, which lower the pH of gastric reflux.

• **Body and fundus** Under the influence of the vagus nerve, they become distended by the ingestion of food. This is where most of the cells secreting pepsinogen, gastric Iipase, intrinsic factor and HCL are found.

• **The antrum and pylorus** These 2 regions act as a kneading trough for the food. The contractions in these areas mix and grind the food before releasing it in small quantities through the pylorus. The pylorus is rich in surface cells, enabling it to reduce the acidity of the chyme it releases into the duodenum (thus protecting the intestinal mucosa from acidity).

> **Gastric secretions :**

Cell types	Main products	Roles
Surface cells	✓ Mucus	✓ Lubrication
Parietal cells	✓ H+	✓ Protein digestion
Main cells	✓ Pepsinogen	✓ Protein digestion
Endocrine cells	✓ Gastrin ✓ Histamine ✓ Somatostatin	✓ Regulation of acid secretion

> **Gastric motility**

When a meal is eaten, the stomach is rapidly distended to accommodate the entire contents of the meal. This distension increases the basic membrane potential of the slow waves (the membrane potential thus approaches the action potential), creating waves of spontaneous contractions with a frequency of around 3/minute. These peristaltic waves travel from the body to the antrum, triggering a pyloric contraction. Since antral pressure only becomes sufficient to overcome pyloric resistance for a short time, the stomach empties by only a few milliliters at a time. The rest of the antral contents then collide with the closed pylorus and rise towards the gastric body like a wave hitting a rock.

3. **The intestinal phase of digestion :**

➢ **Secretions**

The arrival of gastric chyme in the intestine triggers the secretion of several substances by different organs

1) Pancreas: pancreatic secretions

Composition

Pancreatic juice contains high levels of HCO_3^- ions, which, with the help of bile and intestinal secretions, neutralize the pH of the duodenum made acidic by gastric contents. It also contains several enzymes that act on the various components of a meal:

Proteases(Trypsinogen,Chymotrypsinogen,Proelastase, Procarboxypeptidase A, Procarboxypeptidase,

Lipases (Lipase, Phospholipase, Cholesterolesterhydrolase),

Pancreatic amylase, Nucleases (Ribonuclease, Deoxyribonuclease)

2) Gallbladder: bile secretions

Composition

Bile is an aqueous solution containing several solutes, including :

• Bile salts

• Phospholipids

• Cholesterol

• Bilirubin

- HCO3-

- Other electrolytes

Bile salts line up around free fatty acids and cholesterol to form a membrane: micelles.

These micelles carry the lipids to the intestinal brush border, where they are absorbed.

➢ **Intestinal movements**

In addition to peristaltic movement, which helps propel food through the digestive system, the intestine also exhibits segmental contractions, which occur simultaneously at several points in the intestine, giving it a string-like appearance.

4. **The colon**

Since digestion is generally completed higher up in the intestine, the colon plays only a secondary role in this process. Bacteria present in the colon can, however, digest proteins at this level by putrefaction.

Although it is not very active in the digestion of nutrients, the colon nevertheless fulfills several functions:

- Water and ion absorption.

- Bacterial fermentation of unabsorbed nutrients.

- Storage of waste and non-digestible materials.

- Disposal of waste and non-digestible materials.

In order to perform its role as efficiently as possible, the colon reacts to various stimuli:

• **Rectal distension** is perceived and enables the transition between the storage function (muscle relaxation) performed by the colon and the waste excretion function (muscle contraction). This response is made possible by the interaction of the intrinsic and extrinsic nervous systems.

• **A drop in effective circulating volume** leads to increased reabsorption of water and ions via aldosterone.

• **The arrival of free fatty acids in the colon** leads to the release of peptide YY, which inhibits most digestive tract functions, from gastric secretion to colonic motility.

D.   *Digestion and absorption of nutrients*

1. Protein :

Digestion begins in the stomach, thanks to pepsin, and continues in the intestine. Digested proteins come not only from food, but also from enzymes in the intestinal lumen and from cell debris. Digestion of these proteins takes place at 3 levels in the intestine:

• **Intestinal luminosity** thanks to proteolytic enzymes from the pancreas.

Proteins are converted into oligopeptides and a small proportion of amino acids.

• **Brush border** The peptidases of the brush border degrade oligopeptides into dipeptides and tripeptides.

- **Enterocyte cytoplasm** Dipeptides and tripeptides are then hydrolyzed into amino acids in the enterocyte by cytoplasmic peptidase.

Transport of peptides from the intestinal lumen to the cytoplasm of enterocytes :

✓ By a Na+/amino acid cotransporter which internalizes an amino acid together with a Na+ ion

✓ By a Na+/H+ pump that pumps out one H+ for every Na+ that enters the enterocyte. The H+ thus expelled from the cell does not accumulate in the intestinal lumen, as it returns to the enterocyte by electrotraction (the inside of the enterocyte is negative), taking dipeptides and tripeptides with it via a cotransporter.

> ➢ **Absorption**

The vast majority of proteins are absorbed in the duodenum or jejunum. Amino acids and a small quantity of dipeptides and tripeptides leave the enterocyte on the basolateral side and enter the bloodstream via 5 sodium-dependent and sodium-independent transporters.

2. *Glucose :*

- **Intestinal lumen** Starch is transformed into glucose oligomers by salivary and pancreatic amylase.

- **Brush border** Several enzymes act on the different types of sugar to break them down into glucose, fructose or galactose :

Sucrase: breaks down sucrose into glucose and fructose.

Glucoamylase: converts glucose oligomers into glucose.

Lactase: converts lactose into glucose and galactose.

> ### Absorption

A Na+/K+ ATPase pump located on the basal side of the enterocyte brings carbohydrates into the cell.

Na+ carries glucose and galactose with it via several cotransporters. The same applies to the passage of all carbohydrates from the enterocyte to the bloodstream.

Glucose absorption is rapid and complete at the beginning of the small intestine.

3. *Lipids :*

Lipid digestion begins in the mouth and continues in the intestine thanks to pancreatic Iipase.

This acts on TGs to form free fatty acids and 2- monoacylglycerols. These are then internalized in micelles which then transport the lipids to the brush border of the intestine.

Dietary cholesterol and phospholipids are digested by cholesterol ester hydrolase and phospholipase A2 respectively. Their residues are then internalized in micelles that carry them, along with fatty acids and 2-monacylglycerols, to the brush border.

> ### Absorption

Once they reach the brush border, the micelles empty their contents near the apical side of the enterocyte. The lipids then enter the intestinal cells by diffusion. Once inside, cholesterol is re-esterified and fatty acids bind to 2- monoacylglycerols to reform TGs. These two groups of molecules are incorporated into chylomicrons, which enter the lymphatic circulation.

Most lipid absorption takes place in the jejunum and ileum.

4. Water :

➤ Absorption

The total volume of water present in the digestive tract comes from several sources. In addition to oral intake, the intestine receives water from various digestive secretions. Around 98% of the 9 liters of water present in the digestive tract are reabsorbed by the small intestine and colon, leaving just 200 ml of water in the stool.

Water movement in the intestine is determined by the osmotic pressure of the intestinal contents. The body attempts to restore the balance between plasma and intestinal osmolality. The duodenal contents are hyperosmolar, causing a surge of water into the bloodstream which, combined with the influx of digestive secretions, helps to restore equilibrium. As nutrients are absorbed, intestinal osmolality decreases, leading to water reabsorption. This takes place in different ways, depending on the location and conditions in the intestinal lumen:

- **Small intestine :**

Nutrient absorption lowers intestinal osmolality, and water is reabsorbed via the paracellular route.

To achieve this, absorbed glucose stimulates contraction of the actin filaments present in enterocytes. This cellular contraction expands the paracellular zones, facilitating water absorption.

- **Small intestine and colon:**

The absorption of neutral NaCl in the small intestine and colon also reduces intestinal osmolality, leading to water reabsorption.

- **Colon :**

A Na+ pump on the apical side of the enterocyte enables water and other electrolytes to be absorbed paracellularly.

3.2. The Paleolithic or "Paleodiet" diet
A. generality(!)

Hunter-gatherers appear to have been generally healthy, and those who managed to maintain this lifestyle are still in good health. The study of Neolithic skeletons shows a general deterioration in health. And many new "civilization" diseases are appearing with the industrial era and the modern diet, which is moving even further away from the original, natural diet.

In the 1970s, this observation gave rise to the concept of the "*paleo diet*", popularized in the 1980s by Anglo-Saxon dieticians and anthropologists. The radiologist and medical anthropologist S. Boyd Eaton brought this concept to the attention of the media when, in 1985, he published an article entitled "*Paleolithic Nutrition*" in the serious *New England Journal of Medicine.* His theory is that our genes determine our nutritional needs. The human genome is thought to have evolved by only 0.02% over the last 40,000 years, so Paleolithic nutrition would still be perfectly suitable for us. However, this starting point is disputed by some members of the scientific community, as illustrated by a rather critical article published a few days ago in *Le Monde...*

Since 1985, various scientists have been studying this era and determining the dietary practices of Paleolithic hunter-gatherers. One of these researchers, Loren Cordain, a professor in the Department of Health and Exercise Sciences at the University of Colorado, popularized these theses in 2001 in a mainstream book adapted to American culture, *"The Paleo Diet"*, and in the accompanying blog. In it, he describes the prehistoric diet as it should be followed in our time, and has become one of the leaders of the Paleolithic diet. He proposes a return to a diet as close as possible to that of our origins, i.e. the first *homo sapiens* in Europe. The American version of the "Paleolithic diet" does not insist on consuming mostly raw foods, as some of the more crudivorous followers, particularly in Europe, denounce.

In France, this diet has been championed by Thierry Soucar, science journalist and creator of the independent information website *la Nutrition .fr* 168, and by immunonutrition specialist Dr. Dominique Rueffl69 . For the latter, a return to the Paleolithic way of eating - rich in proteins and fiber and low in sugars - can help you lose weight, improve your fitness and health, and prevent a number of serious chronic diseases. This diet is based on strict control of the quantity and quality of carbohydrates ingested, and the eradication of foods for which our digestive and immune physiology is fundamentally unprepared. Traditional cookery books are also available, such as writer

Joseph Delteil's long-standing essay "Paleolithic cuisine"(7).

The Paleolithic diet, which our ancestors practiced for millions of years and to which our physiology is adapted, consisted of game meat and wild plants.

The "paleo diet" is therefore resolutely pre-agricultural, meaning **no salt, sugar, additives or preservatives, but also no cereals or dairy products, based on lean meat or fish, fresh vegetables and fruit.**

B. *Foods for Paleolithic meals and their benefits*

Birds' eggs (or organic hens' eggs) Source of high-quality protein with essential fatty acids in the ideal proportion and carotenoids (lutein, zeaxanthin, beta-carotene), a major source of phosphatidylcholine, precursor of acetylcholine (memory neurotransmitter).

Game reindeer, fallow deer, roe deer, bison, bull, ostrich, kid The flesh of wild or free-range animals is less fatty than that of farmed animals, and richer in omega 3. Long bones provide marrow, rich in phospholipids.

Small game pheasant, quail, woodcock, guinea fowl, hare: contain proteins and sulfur-containing amino acids, precursors of glutathione (the main cellular detoxifier). Cartilage provides silica, glucosamine and chondroitin, which help prevent osteoarthritis.

Small animals snails, frogs, small reptiles: A wealth of amino acids that are precursors of growth hormone: arginine, ornithine, glutamine.

Offal is concentrated with beneficial vitamins and minerals if it comes from free-range animals that have not been treated with medication. Liver is an unrivalled source of vitamin A and vitamin B9, which prevents foetal malformations and reduces cardiovascular risk and

Alzheimer's disease.

Shellfish, oily fish, eels; valuable source of long-chain fatty acids (EPA, DHA) and high-quality proteins, essential minerals: zinc, copper, iron, selenium...

Grasshoppers, crickets, termites, scorpions, beetles, red ants, crickets, caterpillars, silkworm larvae, wasp larvae... High nutritional value: 100 grams of beautiful grasshoppers provide as much protein as the same amount of beef, for only 6 grams of fat! Termites provide 35 milligrams of iron per 100 grams!

Fats Flaxseed and rapeseed oils provide the main fatty acids - oleic, linoleic and alpha-linolenic - in proportions close to those found in the Paleolithic era (although they didn't exist back then).

Cashew nuts, macadamia nuts, Brazil nuts, hazelnuts, almonds, chestnuts provide calcium, fiber, omega-3 and phytosterols(7) Fruits figs, cherries, bananas, mangoes, medlars, pears, apples, plums, grapes, peaches... rich in phenols and cyclic compounds that protect the body from free radicals, minerals that regulate the cardiovascular system (calcium and potassium) Spices dill, anise, star anise, cinnamon, cardamom, turmeric, coriander, cumin... Unsurpassed for their terpene and phenol antioxidant content.

Blackberries, bilberries, strawberries, raspberries, blackcurrants, elderberries, hawthorn berries, rosehips...Source of flavonoids, organic acids (chlorogenic and ellagic acids), Coumarins with antioxidant and detoxifying properties by inducing phase 2 enzymes, which neutralize carcinogenic compounds in food.

Tubers and vegetables onions, garlic, wild artichokes, wild carrots, cabbages of all kinds Paleolithic man scoured the earth for onions and tubers - eaten raw or cooked - which provide sulfur compounds, organic acids, saponins and carotenoids (which the body uses for cell maintenance), as well as glucosinolates, isothiocyanates and indoles, which help protect against toxic substances and stabilize chromosomes.

Wild herbs and plants: amaranth, mugwort, wild chicory, wild asparagus, burdock, watercress, wild spinach, wild fennel, lamb's lettuce, mallow, nettle, sorrel, dandelion, purslane, rocket, meadow salsify, sage, thyme, chervil... can be prepared in salads, soups or decoctions, and contain flavonoids (quercetin, apigenin, catechin, etc.) with antioxidant and antiaggregant properties (reducing capillary fragility and permeability). These herbs also provide carotenoids and terpenes, whose anti-cancer properties are being explored.

Fir, spruce, lime, beech and maple leaves contain chlorophyll and carotenoids. Primrose, violet, marigold, nasturtium, zucchini, borage and acacia flowers... contain mainly antioxidant polyphenols (flavones, flavonol glucosides). Can be added to salads, cooked like spinach, candied or used as a decoction.

Wild mushrooms rich in carotenoids (yellow-orange pigments with antioxidant properties).

This list is not exhaustive, but it gives an idea of the nutrient richness of traditional natural foods. However, it's not easy to eat this kind of food in today's cities.... fl it's obvious that in the West we can no longer follow an authentic prehistoric diet, as the foods of the time (game and non-domesticated plants) are either unavailable or too far removed from modern tastes, but the American paleo diet proposes to draw inspiration from them to approach the nutritional characteristics of the hunter-gatherer diet with today's foods.

C. Loren Cordain's "paleodiet" (7)

1. Foods that hunter-gatherers don't eat

a. cereals and dairy products are far less interesting in terms of vitamins, minerals and phytochemicals than portions of seafood, lean meats, fresh fruit and vegetables providing the same amount of calories. When cereals and dairy products are included in the diet, the result is a nutritionally less dense diet.

b. dairy products and milk in particular (whole, skimmed or fermented) strongly stimulate insulin secretion and promote insulin resistance in children, while increasing a growth factor called IGF-I, which is a risk factor for many epithelial cancers (7)

c. Wheat increases intestinal permeability, which promotes low-noise inflammation that stimulates the development of cardiovascular disease, cancer and autoimmune disorders. As Dr Fasano puts it, the introduction of gluten-containing cereals into the human diet some 10,000 years ago probably represents an "evolutionary mistake" that created the conditions for the development of diseases associated with gluten exposure.

d. Salt We need less than 2g a day, and should not exceed 6g. Today, we consume much more salt, often without realizing it, as it is added to all industrial preparations, even sweetened ones. When ingested in quantities that exceed our capacity to eliminate it, it leads to hypertension (obesity) and could aggravate osteoporosis.

e. Fast sugars and refined flours are not natural foods; they cause obesity, diabetes and acidification of the body, with consequences for joints and bones (arthritis, athritis pain...).

2. The health benefits of a paleo diet today(?)

A "modern" Paleo diet would be more effective than the Mediterranean diet in improving blood lipids and other important health parameters. For Prof. Bernard Jacotot (Hôpital Henri Mondor, Créteil, Val-de-Marne), the Paleolithic diet is well worth its current rehabilitation. *"Fat intake is low, which is compatible with the prevention of coronary heart disease and obesity. Fruits, vegetables and nuts provide fiber, which also contributes to lipid balance. Flour products are limited, which is a good thing, as their complex carbohydrates have glycemic indexes that are too high.* Several recent studies have also concluded that it improves the health of diabetic patients.

-It can also improve or prevent certain autoimmune diseases. More and more scientists agree that leaky gut is a universal trigger of food-borne autoimmunity.

-Many elements of the Western diet increase intestinal permeability: lectins, saponins, gliadin, alcohol, capsaicin, thaumatin- like178 proteins. The paleo diet avoids foods that contribute to these permeability factors (wheat, cereals, pulses, capsaicin-rich chillies) and other foods associated with autoimmune diseases, such as dairy products(7).

a. The abundant **fiber** in this ¾ plant-based diet is one of the keys to good health.

Insoluble fibers such as cellulose (wholegrain cereals, vegetables, etc.) ensure good intestinal transit.

soluble fibers (fruit pectin, seaweed alginates, vegetable gums, etc.) absorb water in the digestive tract to form gels that slow gastric emptying, provide early satiety and slow the rate of absorption of carbohydrates and lipids in the small intestine, thus sparing insulin secretion. They also prevent colon cancer.

-The high protein and dietary fiber content of the Paleo diet quickly provides a feeling of **satiety**, thus preventing snacking and weight gain. One of the aims of this diet is **to achieve long-term weight loss** and better health. It's effective because the elimination of modern foods removes most of the causes of overweight. The only book on the subject by biologist Nancy Cattan is *Maigrir avec le régime Paléo(T)*.

In addition to rapid weight loss, the benefits of "paleodiet" include less fatigue, more energy, fewer digestive problems and allergies (lactose, gluten, etc.), and better prevention of sedentary lifestyle-related illnesses (cardiovascular disease, hypertension, obesity, etc.)180. American enthusiasts interviewed by the *Washington Post* 181 and the *New York Times182* are very convinced and involved in this new lifestyle and diet, which they say they can no longer live without.

3. Disadvantages of this diet

It requires great discipline and self-control, as the dietary restrictions are major. Eliminating 10,000 years of cereal-first eating habits is no easy task. The obstacle is mainly psychological. The sheer number of forbidden foods can tip you into a period of excess that's hard to control. The monotony of the diet is an inconvenience for our age, which is accustomed to diversity and sweetness, and can lead to long-term fatigue. *"Paleo eaters sometimes indulge in a few deviations, often involving chocolate, in order to better cope psychologically with such a diet"* (7).

-For the nutritionist who describes this diet on the Passeportsanté website. *"This diet is far removed from our eating habits, and the pleasure of eating can be completely overshadowed"* (7).

-On the other hand, if we follow this diet without taking care to eat a wide variety of foods, as our ancestors did, nutritional deficits are to be feared. However, some followers eat a lot of meat (easier to find than wild plants) while adopting a pseudo-prehistoric lifestyle with exercises inspired by that era (7).

This "paleodiet" is very expensive for the nature-hungry American city dwellers who practice it regularly (food expenditure estimated at around $70 a day!), and the food is hard to find in the usual commercial circuits. Wild or low-fat meats are too rare to be eaten only by a small number of well-to-do, highly motivated individuals.

-Paleodiete practitioners therefore most often use foods derived from agriculture and animal husbandry - i.e. Neolithic culture - as it is no longer possible to live by hunting and gathering in our Western countries. And eating a lot of fatty farmed meats is not at all conducive to good health, as we'll explain later.

-Fresh plants are not available all year round in our climates, unless they have to travel a lot, which is not at all Paleolithic! And the number of plant species on sale is currently too small for the diversity we need to cover our nutrient requirements.

-True Paleolithic behavior, which consists of eating what nature provides according to the seasons, is impossible to reproduce today in our latitudes, as we are not used to long periods of deprivation. The actual practice of this diet remains fairly limited to a few wealthy originals who are bucking the vegetarian trend.

CHAPTER 4: FOOD GEOGRAPHY

4.1. General

Food geography is a branch of human geography that is still in its infancy. There are undoubtedly many product monographs, and agrarian geography, with the two masterworks by D. Faucher and Pierre Gourou and the many regional monographs, has reached a stage of maturity, but these two aspects of food geography are only two aspects of production: the mode of production and production itself. Product consumption, another fundamental element of food geography, has been only partially analyzed in recent years (11).

A. *Definition of a diet.*

A diet is defined both quantitatively and qualitatively, but to better understand the nuances, it's worth recalling a few details about the three basic elements of our diet: carbohydrates, proteins and lipids.

The food products consumed by human beings contain three kinds of energy substances: carbohydrates, composed of carbon, hydrogen and oxygen, such as sugar, honey, fruit, cereal flours, tubers, roots, etc; lipids or fats (fresh butter, margarine, lard, vegetable oils), with a similar composition but higher energy content, containing 85-99% lipids; proteins, with a more complex chemical composition (carbon, hydrogen, oxygen, nitrogen), since they contain the nitrogen that carbohydrates and lipids lack. . These proteins do not exist in their pure state, but come either from animal products (meat, eggs, milk, fish) or plant products (cereals and legumes). In addition to foods that are required for one element (carbohydrate, lipid or protide), there is a whole range of products that can provide the individual with two or even three. Chocolate provides both carbohydrates and lipids; pulses, carbohydrates and protids; meat and milk are complete foods, particularly milk, whose proportion of carbohydrates, lipids and protids is remarkably balanced.

A few more observations on these three basic elements are in order before we turn to the very definition of a diet. On average, a gram of carbohydrates provides 4.2 calories, a gram of lipids 9.8 and a gram of proteins 4.8, but only proteins contain nitrogenous substances. It follows from these observations that lipids are far superior to carbohydrates and proteins in terms of calories, and that proteins are superior to the other two in terms of nitrogenous matter. The respective share of carbohydrates, lipids and proteins in a diet can therefore be used as a classification criterion.

1. Quantitative definition.

A diet is defined quantitatively by the total number of calories and the percentage of calories from the three basic elements: carbohydrates, fats and proteins.

In the USA, the average diet is 3,250 calories, 55.4% of which are carbohydrates, 19.9% fat and 24.6% protein; in Korea, the average diet is 1,900 calories, 90.4% of which are carbohydrates, 3.7% fat and 5.8% protein.

These two "extreme" examples give rise to two quantitative findings. The total number of calories in an average diet varies between 1,800 and 3,300 calories in different countries; the proportion of carbohydrates varies between 90% and 50%, decreasing as the average diet rises.

But this quantitative definition is incomplete. It does not take into account the extreme variety of food quality within the three main groups of carbohydrates, fats and proteins, the proportion of vitamins, initial calories and final calories - all qualitative notions that are indispensable for a complete definition of a diet and for a classification based on rational criteria.

1. Qualitative definition.

The quantitative definition of a diet must be backed up by other qualitative data: the variety of foods within each group, initial and final calories, vitamins and minerals.

Variety of food quality within each group 2.

Within each group - carbohydrates, fats and proteins - there can be considerable differences between the foods we eat.

Among carbohydrates, "we can distinguish between rich carbohydrates supplied by sugars, and poor carbohydrates from cereals, roots and tubers.

In Denmark, sugar carbohydrates account for 66% of total carbohydrates consumed. It is 62% in Sweden, 52% in the UK, while it is less than 5% in most of Africa and Asia (except in sugarcane-growing areas); 1% in Madagascar, 4% in Kenya, Siam and Indochina, and 1-2% in China.

Calculations based on averages have shown that the share of sugars in total carbohydrate consumption rises progressively from the 1,800-

calorie diet to the 3,000-calorie diet. From 7% in the former case, it rises to 30% in the latter.

Lipids offer an identical variety. Just as there are poor and rich carbohydrates, so a distinction between free and bound lipids can be justified. In fact, lipids can be found either in the pure lipid group (butter, lard, vegetable oils), in which case they are usually referred to as free lipids, or in a more complex group of foods providing carbohydrates and proteins at the same time, in which case they are referred to as bound lipids. A higher consumption of free lipids indicates a higher standard of living and a more advanced diet.

In the USA, where the average diet exceeds 3,200 calories, lipid consumption is 140 g per person per day, and 49.6% comes from free lipids. In Japan, where the average diet for the period 1936-1938 was 2,200 calories, lipid consumption was only 24.5 g per person per day, and free lipids accounted for only 19%.

Average calculations revealed the following observations: as the diet becomes richer, lipid consumption rises: total lipids increase by 21%, free lipids by 29% and bound lipids by 18%, each time the diet increases by around a hundred calories a day. On average, the percentage of free lipids rises from 30% for a low-calorie diet (2,000 calories per day) to 39% for a high-calorie diet (3,000 calories).

Proteins also differ in quality. Animal proteins (meat, eggs, milk, fish) are far superior to plant proteins. The more advanced the diet, the higher the protein intake, but the lower the proportion of plant-based proteins. For example, in Sweden (period 1934-1938), for an average diet of

3,050 calories, protide consumption per person per day was 88 g, of which 62% was of animal origin. By contrast, in China, where the average diet was 2,200 calories, the consumption of protein from pulses was 68g, of which only 7% was of animal origin.

So there are rich carbohydrates and poor carbohydrates, noble proteins and ordinary proteins, pure or free lipids and bound lipids. Clearly, an advanced diet is characterized not only by an increase in the number of calories, but also by a decrease in the percentage of poor carbohydrates and proteins of plant origin, and an increase in free lipids and proteins of animal origin.

This extreme variety within the three major groups enables us to establish certain criteria for differentiating diets. But they need to be supplemented by two other concepts, in particular the ratio of initial calories to final calories (12).

2. Initial and final calories.

When cereals are consumed directly by humans, the number of calories absorbed, or final calories, is equal to the number of initial calories. On the other hand, when cereals, roots and tubers are consumed by animals, it takes around seven calories to restore one of them in the form of meat or milk. In this case, the number of final calories is seven times less than the number of initial calories.

Thus, the consumption of animal products (indirect consumption) requires far more calories than that of plant products (direct consumption). But, in a twist of fate, these calories are more valuable: the initial calories were essentially made up of poor carbohydrates, whereas the final calories are rich in proteins and lipids.

Ultimately, the ratio of initial calories to final calories can vary from 3 to 1, depending on the level of diet.

3. Vitamins and minerals.

A diet would not be completely defined if it were not characterized by the presence or deficiency of vitamins and minerals. Let's recall very briefly that vitamins can be classified into two categories: some are water-soluble, found in the aqueous fraction of plants, while others are iiposoluble, found in certain fat constituents.

Among the first, the B and C complex vitamins seem fundamental. Vitamin Bl is anti-neurotic; its deficiency leads to nervous disorders and plays a key role in the development of the dreaded beriberi disease; rice is virtually devoid of this vitamin. Growth vitamin B2 is found in most plant and animal products. On the other hand, vitamin PP, which is lacking in a widespread food such as corn, plays a considerable role, since its deficiency leads to pellagra. Vitamin G, which is essentially antiscorbutic, is commonly found in fresh vegetables, especially oranges and lemons.

Among the ranks of Iiposoluble vitamins, vitamin A seems essential, since its deficiency leads to visual problems, mucous membrane lesions and reduced muscle tone. It is derived from the oxidation of carotene, and is found in fish oils and liver, butter, certain vegetable oils, certain yellow fruits and carrots. Vitamin D plays an anti-rachitic role, while vitamin E can be considered the reproductive vitamin.

Finally, the mineral salts essential to a good diet are those that provide calcium, phosphorus, iron and iodine, a deficiency of which can lead to nervous disorders.

A diet is defined by the total number of calories, by the respective share of carbohydrates, lipids and proteins in calorie production, by the variety and composition of foods within each group, by the number of initial calories and final calories, and possibly by vitamin or mineral deficiencies.

It's easy to see how difficult and complex a classification would be. Careful analysis of these five data leads us to propose an initial distinction between simple and complex diets.

4.2. Simple diets.

These are diets comprising a small number of products and characterized by one or two predominant staple foods. They generally characterize countries where foreign trade involves only a very small number and small quantity of agricultural products. They are the lot of peoples with an agricultural or pastoral economy, while complex diets are associated with a more industrial economy. But they affect very different countries, some overpopulated like those of Monsoon Asia, others sparsely populated like those of South America. These regions can be very poor in calories, as in Asia, or very rich (Argentina, Uruguay). That's why it's essential to distinguish between primitive and simple, richer diets.

A) Primitive regimes.

A primitive diet. It is characterized by a calorie count of less than 2,500, which can be considered a maximum, with an average of between 1,900 and 2,300 calories. It is also characterized by an animal protein intake of less than 15g per person per day, and a lipid intake of less than 50g per person per day. But the dominant feature of this diet is the predominance of carbohydrates, over 80%, and the very low proportion (under 15%) of expensive carbohydrates derived from sugar as a proportion of total carbohydrates. Two other criteria help to define this diet even more fully: the loss between initial and final calories is always less than 50% and, finally, this low-carbohydrate diet, with rice and corn predominating, may be deficient in vitamins B 1, PP, A and D and in mineral salts.

Geographic expansion.

This primitive diet affects more than half of humanity, and extends over vast regions of Asia, Africa and South America. In Asia, China (2,130 calories), Japan and India (2,021), Indochina (2,127), Java (2,040), the Philippines, Malaysia, Siam, Burma and Ceylon all meet these criteria. In South America, Peru, Bolivia and Colombia also fall into this food category, and certain sectors of Brazil and Chile should also be included. In Africa, studies show that Egypt, Madagascar and Kenya have an average primitive diet.

B. Richer simple diets.

These are diets whose total calorie count, reaching or exceeding 2,500, is higher than that of primitive diets, but which remain simple because they are made up of a small number of foods. The main difference with primitive diets lies in the lower proportion of poor carbohydrates, always less than 80%, and the existence of one or more rich foods (rich carbohydrates, lipids or proteins) in appreciable quantities. These simple diets can themselves be grouped into large families.

Firstly, we can distinguish diets with a high proportion of rich carbohydrates, i.e. sugar. These generally correspond to the major sugarcane-growing areas of the West Indies, certain parts of India (Ganges plain) and Brazil. The proportion of sugar is always higher than 20% of total carbohydrates, whereas it never reached 15% in primitive diets.

A second type is represented by the high proportion of lipids, particularly free lipids, i.e. derived directly from fats. In these diets, the proportion of lipids is generally higher than that of proteins, and the proportion of free lipids exceeds 45% of total lipids. This is essentially the diet of Mediterranean countries, a simple diet based on cereals and olive oil. Spain and Greece are perhaps the two Mediterranean peninsulas that offer the best example. In Spain, where the average diet amounts to 2,788 calories (74% carbohydrates, 13.4% lipids and 12.5% proteins), the proportion of free lipids is 48%. In Greece, where the average diet is 2,523 calories, carbohydrates make up 71.1%, lipids 17.8% and proteins 11%; the proportion of free lipids is 61%, the highest in the world. In addition to Spain and Greece, which are highly representative of this type of diet, Portugal, Italy, Algeria, Tunisia and Palestine also belong to this group. All these countries have a predominantly cereal-based agricultural system, and many practice biennial fallowing or dry-farming (large estates belonging to latifundia or North African European farms). Livestock farming therefore plays a secondary role, while olive groves have been part of the rural landscape since antiquity.

In a third type, the rich element is represented by proteins. This simple diet, based on cereals and meat, characterizes all the major livestock-producing countries: Southern Brazil (Rio Grande state), Uruguay, Paraguay, Argentina). The number of calories is much higher, almost always exceeding 2,800; the proportion of protein exceeds 30% and that of animal protein reaches or exceeds 60%. Of course, the number of initial calories is very high compared to the number of final calories, and wastage exceeds 65%. Two examples, Argentina and Uruguay, are highly illustrative. In Argentina, where the average diet amounts to 3,200 calories, the proportion of carbohydrates is only 59%, while the proportion of protein is 33.5% (of which 58% is animal protein). The example of Uruguay is perhaps even more significant: the total number of calories is 2,900, the proportion of carbohydrates 56.9%, that of proteins 39.1%, of which 62% are animal proteins (the highest proportion in the world after Australia, equivalent to that of Sweden and Iceland).

This diet is easily explained. Uruguay, Argentina and southern Brazil are major livestock-producing countries, and the farming system, often very simple, consists of more or less prolonged alternation of alfalfa fields and cereals. A diet based on wheat and meat seems the logical consequence of this type of agricultural economy.

Finally, a fourth type of simple but rich diet is that of the Eskimos or Lapps, who make their living from fishing, hunting or reindeer husbandry, fl characterized by a very high proportion of lipids and protids and a low share of carbohydrates.

All these simple diets, whether primitive or richer, can be found in countries of very old civilization (Monsoon Asia or the Mediterranean basin) or in the new countries of temperate South America. On the other hand, in most countries of Western civilization, diets are much more complex.

4.3. Complex diets.

Complex diets are characterized by a much greater variety of foods, by the richness of these foods and by their higher cost. While there are, as in the diets previously studied, a few staple foods, the proportion of carbohydrates, lipids and protids is achieved by a much more complex interplay involving cereals, free fats, animal protids, vegetables, fruit, eggs, fish, dairy products, sugar, cocoa, etc., etc., etc., etc. These complex diets offer common geographical features that do not exclude variety.

A.   *Common geographical features.*

These are the diets of white peoples, especially those of Western civilization. North America (U.S.A. and Canada), Oceania (Australia and New Zealand), Western Europe (France, U.K., Belgium, Netherlands, Federal Republic of Germany, Switzerland, Austria), Scandinavia (Norway, Sweden, Denmark, Iceland, Finland) undoubtedly have average diets meeting these criteria. The countries of Central and Eastern Europe (Poland, Hungary, Romania, Bulgaria, U.S.S.R.) can be considered, because of their highly cereal-based character, as a transition region between countries with simple and complex diets.

In fact, these complex diets are defined by their high calorie count (2,800 to 3,200 calories), by the much lower proportion of carbohydrates (below 70%, and as low as 50.7% in New Zealand), and by the high percentage of rich carbohydrates, i.e. sugar as a proportion of total carbohydrates, which always exceeds 30% and can even rise to 66%, as in Denmark. The proportion of animal protein always exceeds 35% of total protein, reaching 60% in Scandinavian countries. Final calories compared to initial calories always represent a loss of over 50%, and in some cases as much as 75%. Finally, foods that are not usually considered staples - fruit, citrus fruit, a wide variety of green vegetables - play a much more important role than in previous diets.

These complex diets correspond to regions of the world where the agricultural system combines livestock farming with crop rotation. They are also part of a trading economy, involving the import of a wide range of food products and the export of cereals to overpopulated countries, or of industrial products to under-equipped countries. Ultimately, these complex food regimes correspond to the great industrialized zone of the world, which encompasses North America and Europe, and which is also the great zone that developed the agricultural and livestock revolution during the XfXth and XXth centuries.

Finally, these complex diets affect countries which, to a greater or lesser extent, have practised Malthusianism: fairly low natural growth, very moderate birth rates. On the other hand, these are countries with average or low rural densities; high human densities are localized, with the possible exception of the Netherlands, in industrial and urban sectors.

However, uniformity is far from the rule here, and three variants can be distinguished: diets with a high percentage of cereals, a high percentage of dairy products and a high percentage of meat.

B. The cereal type.

Some countries with complex, varied and rich diets continue to consume large quantities of cereals, with annual per capita consumption exceeding 100 kg. In addition to the countries of Central and Eastern Europe, which are heavy consumers of cereals and hardly deserve to be classed as regions with complex diets, France, Ireland and, to a lesser degree, Germany and Switzerland are in this group. This is largely due to the system of land ownership (small and medium-sized farmers) and the large proportion of Fauto-Consumption; on the other hand, France is a nation of peasants, where even city dwellers have a peasant origin, and therefore eating habits inherited from generations of peasants for whom bread held a large place in daily food.

C. Diets with a high percentage of woollens.

These diets are particularly prevalent in Scandinavia (Norway, Sweden, Denmark), New Zealand, the UK, the USA, the Netherlands and Switzerland. Per capita milk consumption per year exceeds 240 kg everywhere, while in France it is just 160 kg. The maximum is Norway (340 kg per year), while consumption is still ? 240 kg in the U.S.A., and over 300 kg in Switzerland, Sweden, Denmark and New Zealand.

These diets, in which dairy products are given pride of place, correspond for the most part to large livestock-raising countries, but where farming is geared more towards the production of milk, butter and cheese than meat, unlike South American countries which are larger producers of meat than milk. Moreover, this orientation of livestock farming corresponds to Western and Nordic peoples' tastes for fresh butter and cheese, and to a type of intensive livestock farming.

D.   *Meat-based diets.*

Australia in particular, with a consumption of 108 kg per capita per year, falls into this category; only Uruguay has a higher consumption. In fact, this diet is similar to that of South American countries with extensive livestock farming and cereal crops, also extensive; however, a higher average standard of living and Anglo-Saxon eating habits introduce a greater variety of foods.

We have just attempted to classify diets. We make no secret of the imperfections of this classification which, like all such attempts, is too systematic. At the very least, it enables us to highlight the links that exist between diets and certain determining geographical factors.

4.4. Diets and the geographical phenomena that determine them.

In our previous sections, in trying to explain the different types of diet, we have highlighted the role of agricultural or farming systems, the influence of social structures or demographic phenomena, depending on the case. The time has now come to bring these observations together to identify the fundamental links between diets and geographical phenomena. This essay highlights the predominant role of climate, which partly controls agricultural systems and farming methods. Social, political and economic factors also play a decisive role. Finally, this review would be incomplete without highlighting the interdependence of diets and demographic regimes.

A. *The predominant role of climate.*

Climate has a fundamental influence on basic metabolism and on the quality of food adapted to the organism, depending on whether it lives in a polar or tropical climate. The following conclusions can be drawn from the numerous, often contradictory, studies carried out on basic metabolism.

Cold climates stimulate people to exercise to combat the cold. As a result, the basic metabolism is increased, appetite aroused, and the consumption of fats becomes a necessity. Fats are used more quickly than other foods to form or renew the fat cushion essential to protect against the cold. On the other hand, cold climates whet the appetite, and the fats lining the gastric mucosa give a feeling of sufficiency that a copious, rich ration of other, too-quickly-digested foods would not maintain long enough. These findings help to justify the meat-and-fat diet of the Eskimos and Lapps.

Contrary to long-held beliefs, hot climates produce a higher basal metabolic rate than temperate climates: physical effort requires greater energy expenditure, and recovery times are much longer. On the other hand, hot climates are responsible for a lack of appetite and difficult digestion* of highly concentrated fats (oils, Brazil nuts in the Amazon, where the fat concentration reaches 68%). The difficulty of the effort calls for a very rich diet, including lipids and proteins, but which is not too concentrated and is enhanced by certain peppers needed to stimulate the appetite. These observations prove that the average diet practised in most tropical countries is ill-adapted.

Temperate climates appear to be the most favorable for human nutrition. Basic metabolism is lower here than in cold and hot climates, and the climate allows for a wide variety of crops, making this the climatic zone for rich, complex diets.

This example shows that climate has a decisive influence not only on basic metabolism, but above all on agricultural systems.

4.5. The fundamental role of agricultural systems and farming methods.

Farming systems and farming methods play a decisive role in determining diets.

A. Farming systems.

The slash-and-burn system with long forest fallow practised in some parts of Indochina, Africa and America is a primitive agricultural system. In general, the soil is entrusted with several types of seeds or tubers. This results in a main crop, which provides carbohydrates, and accessory crops (groundnuts, beans, yams, etc.). After two or three years of cultivation, five at most, the field is abandoned and returned to the forest or savannah.

What impact does this farming system have on diets? On the one hand, it doesn't combine livestock farming with cultivation at all; on the other hand, it is practised in areas of Africa, America and Asia where the livestock trade is very important.

Finally, as a result of the long forest fallow periods and primitive farming methods, a large surface area is required per inhabitant, and densities are often higher than optimum. All in all, this agricultural system generates a primitive diet.

The more advanced fallow system is found on large estates in Spain, Portugal and North Africa, as well as on some of the most drought-stricken farms in the Middle West, the Canadian Prairies and Australia. In general, cereal crops alternate with fallow.

This cereal-based system gives limited space to livestock when the fallow is not ploughed, and none at all when the fallow is ploughed. On the other hand, it affects today's most modern and mechanized countries (North America, Australia), as well as old civilizations where fallowing is a survival of the past (latifundia of the Mediterranean peninsulas). In the former case, it has no impact on diets; in the latter, it calls on an abundant workforce and imposes a simple diet based on carbohydrates and olive oil (as a supplement).

The system of continuous cultivation based on human labor is an agricultural system in which the land does not rest, but is improved by human labor. It is practiced today in China, Japan, Indochina and India; the continuous crop is rice, which may alternate with a dry crop during the same growing season. This system is associated with very high population density, resulting in extremely fragmented plots. Animal husbandry is excluded. The result is a primitive diet based on poor carbohydrates.

Continuous cropping with crop rotation is the only system that combines livestock farming with agriculture, and crop rotation with artificial grassland can vary ad infinitum. This system is therefore linked to rich or complex diets. This is the system found in most of the temperate zone of Europe and North America.

Farming systems have a direct impact on diet. The same applies to farming methods.

B.   *Operating modes.*

Colonial-style farming is represented by sugarcane plantations in the West Indies and N.E. Brazil, coffee plantations in the State of Saint Paul, and peanut, cocoa and rubber plantations in Africa, America and Malaysia. These farms are characterized by export-oriented cultivation and the use of cheap labor. They often lead to rapid soil exhaustion, and risk ruining regional subsistence farming for many years to come. While this type of farming helps to generate foreign currency earnings in some countries, it generally leads to an immediate dietary deficiency among agricultural workers, who make up the bulk of the population.

The large mechanized farms of North America employ relatively few people. This type of farming has no direct impact on diets. It contributes indirectly to improving diets through the role played by large-scale mechanized farms in national agriculture.

Small farms are more widespread in Europe and especially in Monsoon Asia. They may be owned by the peasant who works them (which is almost the case in Europe), or by merchants who have invested the profits from their trade in the purchase of land, or who have simply appropriated the land of their debtors (common examples in Japan, China and South-East Asia in general).

These small farms are essentially food crops. They are often too small to be able to rotate crops rationally, and livestock farming is necessarily of secondary importance. The result is a rather poor diet for the smallholder himself, who has no cash at his disposal. From a national perspective, small-scale farming is not always beneficial to agricultural production, and yields are often very low. Indirectly, it does not contribute to raising the level of the diet.

The medium-sized rural farm appears particularly favorable. Properly managed, it can enable rational crop rotation, the development of a cash crop in addition to food crops, the combination of livestock farming and agriculture, and very satisfactory yields thanks to the intensive and meticulous nature of the cultivation. It is adapted to medium rural densities. Essentially European, it is linked to a rich and complex diet.

In short, slash-and-burn shifting cultivation, continuous cultivation based on human labor on very small farms, colonial-style cultivation and exploitation, and latifundia practicing fallowing are not conducive to a high average diet. On the other hand, farming systems with crop rotation, which combine livestock and agriculture on either medium-sized or large mechanized farms, raise the average diet. Farming systems and farming methods reflect social, economic and political structures.

4.6. Social, economic and political structures.

Insofar as national or regional agricultural production is insufficient to ensure a suitable diet, its improvement is linked to the general economy, export or import possibilities, transport, international aid and economic agreements.

On the other hand, social factors seem easier to determine. The existence of two distinct social classes, one rich and one poor, is not conducive to a high average diet. The example of Monsoon Asia and many South American countries is quite evocative. On the contrary, the existence of a developed middle class is conducive to a rich, well-balanced average diet. This is the case in most of Europe and North America. Clearly, the map of primitive diets coincides with that of a two-class social structure and the non-existence of a middle class (in India, the middle class constitutes barely 2.5% of the population). On the contrary, the map of rich diets corresponds to the geographical expansion of a large middle class, the result of the agricultural and industrial revolution that took place at the end of the 19th century among peoples of European civilization.

Even more instructive is the superimposition of the map of diets and demographic regimes.

4.7. Diets and demographic regimes.

Josué de Castro may have written, at the head of a book, this popular saying: "The poor man's table is meager, but the bed of misery is fertile". No doubt this is a rather spectacular presentation of the links between diets and demographic regimes, but these links are undeniable, as demonstrated by the simultaneous analysis of primitive diets and demographic regimes, and of complex diets and mature demographic regimes.

A. Primitive diets and demographic regimes.

Primitive diets are in fact linked to primitive demographic regimes. Undernourished countries all have high birth rates. Rates are above 30%0 everywhere in Monsoon Asia, Central and South America, and in most Mediterranean countries (40%0 in China, 33%0 in India, 40%o in Egypt). Similarly, undernourished peoples have very high mortality rates (average rates over 20%0, 27%o in Egypt, 25%0 in India, 30%o in China). Infant mortality rates oscillate between 150 and 200 %0 (N.E. Brazil). What's more, in these countries with primitive diets, mortality rates are very high in the 15-20 age bracket, as people make the transition from adolescence to adulthood. The result is a very high percentage of under-20s, and a low percentage of adults.

Very high natural growth in excess of 10%0 is therefore the result of primitive diets, which are also primitive demographics.

* Birth and death rates have been calculated for a 15-year average according to the United Nations Demographic Yearbook.

B.   Complex diets and mature demographic regimes.

Conversely, countries with complex diets are also Malthusian countries. They correspond to a higher standard of living and the development of a larger middle class, birth rates are generally moderate, below 20%0, and above all mortality rates are much lower (between 8% and 1%0). Infant mortality rates are below 80%0, and life expectancy is higher. The structure of the population is completely different: the percentage of adults is much higher (between 50 and 55%), whereas it oscillated between 43 and 47% among peoples with primitive demographic regimes, who are also the sojus-alimented peoples.

The example of Brazil is a remarkable illustration of this dual comparison between primitive diets and primitive demographic regimes, on the one hand, and complex diets and evolved demographic regimes, on the other. It also illustrates no less strikingly the opposition between the colonial-style farming system and the European-style agricultural system.

I° Diets are undoubtedly linked to agricultural systems and forms of farming. The combination of agriculture and livestock farming is undoubtedly the agricultural economy that ensures the highest average food level. Colonial-style farming may be useful to a country's economy by providing export products, but in strictly human terms, it is accompanied by an agricultural proletariat, and therefore by a relatively low average food level.

2° The map of diets coincides with that of primitive demographic regimes. The half of humanity that is undernourished is also the half of humanity with the highest birth rates, the highest mortality rates and the greatest natural increase.

3° The undernourished, overpopulated block of Monsoon Asia, with its subsistence agriculture and small rural farms; the tropical countries of Africa and South America, often poorly exploited and therefore undernourished despite low population densities; the temperate countries of the southern hemisphere, characterized by simple but rich diets, linked to an agricultural system in which livestock farming plays a major role; the temperate countries of the northern hemisphere, which in the 19th century underwent the agricultural and industrial revolution, and for the past century have practised colonialism and Malthusianism, now enjoy a rich and complex diet, thanks to rational agriculture and livestock breeding, a trading economy and moderate natural population growth(12).

CHAPTER 5: THE CARNIVOROUS DIET

5.1. Definition

The carnivorous diet is a trend that's all the rage, and many people have reported significant benefits from adopting **an all-meat diet.** But is **eating nothing but meat** healthy in the long term? Read on to understand the mechanisms behind the diet, the potential consequences of not eating plant foods and some alternatives for **becoming a pure carnivore.**

The carnivore diet is quite simple: eat only foods of animal origin and stay away from all plant foods. This means that **your energy comes mainly from proteins and fats**, and that you consume almost zero carbohydrates.

The carnivore diet means completely eliminating plant foods, so no fruits, vegetables, grains, nuts, seeds or legumes. Instead, the approximate list of dietary foods for carnivores looks like this:

- Red meat (especially fatty cuts)

- Offal

- Poultry

- Fish

- Eggs

- Tallow and lard

- Bone broth

- Marrow

Some dieters eat high-fat, low-lactose dairy products such as hard cheeses, heavy cream and butter, while others avoid dairy products altogether. Strict carnivore diets may also eliminate coffee and tea - they are plant-based drinks, after all. Seasonings can also be restricted: salt and pepper are generally allowed, but some dieters won't venture that far.

Many people who have adopted the carnivorous diet report faster weight loss, better mental clarity, healthier digestion and even improved sports performance. I certainly don't doubt the anecdotal reports of people who have found remarkable relief from debilitating chronic health problems with this diet. For many of these people, nothing else has worked.

However, when considering an intervention from a dietary health or lifestyle point of view, I often believe we should look at the bigger picture: historical evidence from other populations, plausible mechanisms that explain its effect on our bodies, and scientific data regarding outcomes.

5.2. Carnivore versus ketogenic diet
What's the **difference between the carnivorous diet and the ketogenic diet?**

Both emphasize fat and protein, but keto allows *some* carbohydrates (albeit a very small amount). While carnivores try to eat as close to zero carbohydrates as possible, the ketogenic diet, which is classified as very low carb, allows 5 to 10% of calories from carbohydrates.

For reference:

• In a low-carb diet, carbohydrates account for 10-15% of total daily calories.

• A moderate carbohydrate diet provides 15 to 30 percent.

• A diet rich in carbohydrates exceeds 30%.

Perhaps the most notable difference is that the restriction of the carnivore diet is not part of keto. While keto followers will probably eat many of the same animal-based foods allowed in the carnivore diet, since they emphasize protein and fat, they can also eat plant-based foods, provided they are low in carbohydrates.

I'll explain the effects and benefits of a ketogenic diet in more detail below, but you can consider a carnivorous diet to be more restrictive and even lower in carbohydrates than keto.

5.3. Ancestral carnivorous populations

A brief overview of the diets of certain ancestral populations claimed to be "carnivores". Indeed, many ancestral groups thrived on large quantities of animal products. However, each of these groups also took advantage of plant foods when they were available:

• Mongolian nomads ate meat and dairy products, but also derived nutrients from wild onions and garlic, tubers and roots, seeds and berries (13).

• Brazilian Gauchos consumed mainly beef, but supplemented their diet with yerba mate, an herbal infusion rich in vitamins, minerals and phytonutrients(14).

• The Maasai, Rendille and Samburu of East Africa consumed mainly meat, milk and blood. Young men ate almost exclusively these animal products, but also occasionally consumed herbs and tree bark. Older men and women ate fruits, tubers and honey (15).

• The Chukotka of the Russian Arctic lived on fish, caribou and marine animals, but always ate them with local roots, leafy vegetables, berries or seaweed (16).

• The Sioux of South Dakota ate large quantities of buffalo meat, but they also ate wild fruits, nuts and seeds they found following the buffalo herds (17).

• The Canadian Inuit lived mainly on walrus, whale meat, seal and fish, but they also went to great lengths to feed on wild berries, lichens and sea vegetables. They even fermented some of these plant foods to preserve them (18).

All the cultures we know and have studied ate a combination of animal and plant foods. This doesn't necessarily mean that animal or plant foods are necessary for good health, but it does testify to the ancient wisdom of these cultures: "Nothing in biology makes sense except in the light of evolution." *Theodosius Dobzhansky.*

For 66,000 generations, humans have eaten a variety of foods such as meat, fish, fruits, vegetables, nuts, seeds and certain starchy plants. Contemporary hunter-gatherers fit this general ancestral pattern, although, as you can see above, there's room for variation. But one key point is true: the ancestral approach to eating emphasizes the foods with which our bodies are adapted to thrive.

The diet that best suits your own body could be higher or lower in carbohydrates, fats or even protein (but perhaps not as high as the carnivore diet). The right diet for each individual depends on his or her health, goals, and the diet and lifestyle that would best serve them basic concepts of functional and ancestral health (19).

5.4. Benefits of a carnivorous diet

When a diet, medication or other intervention "works", it's important to try and understand the mechanism. In the case of the carnivorous diet, there are several possible reasons for the benefits people report.

A. The carnivorous diet can limit calories, mimic fasting and help you lose weight fast

Proteins are very satiating, which means they fill you up and send signals to the brain that you've consumed enough food. It's not surprising that people report not feeling very hungry and start eating less often when they adopt an all-meat diet (20).

Food habituation can also play a role here. When you eat the same thing day after day, your brain doesn't get as much **reward value** from the food, so you start eating less food overall, even if that food is usually something you find rewarding, like a big Steakjuteux.

The ultimate result is **unintentional caloric restriction.** Caloric restriction triggers a number of changes. As caloric intake decreases, the concentration of insulin, insulin-like growth factor 1 (IGF-I) and growth hormone is significantly reduced. This condition triggers autophagy, which literally means "self-feeding" - an internal process of cleaning out old cells and repairing damaged ones. Autophagy is also induced during fasting.

Perhaps this is why caloric restriction is so effective in reducing inflammation and alleviating the symptoms of autoimmune diseases (21). Of course, calorie restriction also leads to weight loss. These are probably the two main reasons why people seem attracted to the carnivore way of eating, but these effects could also be achieved by simple caloric restriction.

B. The carnivorous diet is a low-residue diet

Residues" are essentially undigested foods that make up stool. A low-residue diet is one that limits fiber-rich foods such as whole grains, nuts, seeds, fruits and vegetables. It is often prescribed to people with inflammatory bowel disease or **irritable bowel syndrome** to relieve symptoms such as diarrhea, bloating, gas and abdominal pain.

Meat is mainly composed of proteins and fats, which are absorbed very high up in the gastrointestinal tract, leaving little residue to irritate or inflame the intestine. In other words, an all-meat diet is actually a very low-residue diet and gives the intestine a rest.

C. The carnivorous diet is often ketogenic

If you eat large quantities of meat but only eat once or twice a day and add extra fat to the meat, your diet is probably ketogenic. A ketogenic diet is one that is high in fat and moderate in protein, with :

- 60-70% of energy from fats

- 20-30% energy from protein

- 5 to 10% energy from carbohydrates

Although the carnivorous diet doesn't have such macronutrient ratios, it's likely that some of the benefits of eating meat alone are due to the body being in a state of ketosis.

Ketogenic diets have proved useful for a wide variety of conditions, including multiple sclerosis, diabetes and neurological diseases such as Parkinson's and Alzheimer's (22,23).

D.   ***The carnivorous diet changes the intestinal microbiota***

Switching to an all-meat diet can also rapidly alter gut microbiota. A 2014 study found that placing healthy human volunteers on an animal product diet led to significant changes in gut microbiota within 48 hours (24). The animal-based diet increased the abundance of bile-tolerant organisms and decreased levels of microbes known to metabolize various plant fibers.

The gut microbiota has been linked to virtually every chronic inflammatory disease studied, so it's not surprising that an intervention that radically changes the gut microbiota could have significant health implications(25).

5.5. Nutrient deficiencies
Four micronutrients are particularly difficult to obtain on a meat-only

diet. Based on a typical carnivore diet and the Dietary Reference Intakes (DRI) established by the Institute of Medicine, these include:

- Vitamin C: an antioxidant that stimulates immune cell function and is important for stimulating collagen synthesis

- Vitamin E: an antioxidant that prevents oxidation of lipids and lipoproteins

- Vitamin K2: an insoluble vitamin that reduces the calcification of blood vessels

- Calcium: a mineral needed for healthy bones, muscle contraction and nerve transmission

If dairy products are included in the diet, this will cover vitamin K2 and calcium. However, if you don't like offal, the number of potential micronutrient deficiencies increases considerably.

In this case, you can add :

- Vitamin A: An insoluble vitamin important for good vision and maintaining the immune system

- Folate: B vitamin important for cell growth, metabolism and methylation

- Manganese: A trace element necessary for the proper functioning of the nervous system, collagen formation and protection against oxidative stress.

- Magnesium: a mineral that supports over 300 biochemical

reactions, including energy production, DNA repair and muscle contraction.

It's also important to note that vitamin C is extremely sensitive to heat, so only fresh or very gently cooked offal contains appreciable quantities of the vitamin.

Many carnivores claim that the nutritional requirements of the general population simply don't apply to them. Anecdotally, I know several people who have consumed a carnivorous diet for three years or more without any obvious signs of nutrient deficiency.

Yet we lack data. At present, DRIs are the best we have to get rid of, and I don't think we have enough evidence to say unequivocally that this diet is unlikely to produce nutrient deficiencies in the general population.

5.6. Recommended daily intake

Even if the carnivorous diet were sufficient to avoid outright deficiency, the metabolic reserve would also have to be considered. Metabolic reserve is the capacity of cells, tissues and organ systems to resist repeated changes in physiological needs. In other words, it's having enough nutrients "in the bank" to cope with a major stress factor, injury or environmental exposure (26). So, while a person on an all-meat diet may manage to meet a recommended nutritional intake, this may not be enough for optimal health.

5.7. Possible side effects of an all-meat diet

It lacks beneficial phytonutrients, which support health.

Phytonutrients are chemicals produced by plants to protect themselves against environmental threats, such as insect and disease attacks. They can also have major benefits for our health. Curcumin, beta-carotene, quercetin and resveratrol are all examples of common phytonutrients.

Some proponents of the carnivorous diet suggest that phytonutrients are toxic to humans and best eliminated from our diet altogether. However, many of these "toxins" act as acute stressors that make us stronger through a process called hormesis.

Just as resistance training is an acute stressor that leads our muscles to adapt and become stronger, exposure to small amounts of phytonutrients is a homeotic stressor that activates several different pathways in the body, ultimately serving to reduce inflammation, boost immunity, improve cellular communication, repair DNA damage and even detoxify potential carcinogens (27,28).

A. *Effects on hormones, fertility and thyroid function*

An all-meat, carbohydrate-free diet can have adverse effects on hormones, thyroid function and fertility. Carbohydrates are particularly important for female fertility, and very low-carb diets may not be the best choice during pregnancy .

Carbohydrates are particularly important for supporting thyroid function, as insulin stimulates the conversion of inactive thyroid hormone T4 to active T3. In fact, traditional cultures that ate largely animal products and had little access to plant foods often went to great lengths to support fertility, including eating the thyroid glands of the animals they hunted (28).

B. overload your liver

Insufficient consumption of carbohydrates and fats means that the liver can manufacture glucose from proteins via a process known as neoglucogenesis. This process creates nitrogenous waste, which must be converted into urea and eliminated by the kidneys.

While this is a normal process that occurs in every human being, there's a limit to how much protein the liver can safely handle. More than 35-40% of total calories in the form of protein can overwhelm the urea cycle, leading to nausea, diarrhea, emaciation and, potentially, death. For pregnant women, this threshold can be as low as 25 percent of total calories (29).

Interestingly, anthropological evidence suggests that hunters throughout history avoided consuming excess protein, even rejecting low-fat animals when food was scarce (30).

In short: when you eat meat, it's important to have a good amount of healthy fats and quality carbohydrates.

5.8. Five alternatives to the carnivorous diet

Here are a few options that may offer the same therapeutic benefits as the carnivorous diet, but without as many potential risks.

A. A low-carb paleo diet

Some people who try a carnivore diet go straight from the standard

American diet to pure carnivore. Often, a low-carb Paleo model can offer some of the same benefits, including weight loss, improved insulin sensitivity and relief from autoimmune symptoms (31,32,33).

B. A fasting-like diet

A **fasting-mimicking diet** can reverse type 1 and type 2 diabetes, attenuate age-dependent impairment of cognitive performance, and protect against cancer and aging in mice (34,35,36). In humans, the fasting-mimicking diet has been found to significantly reduce body weight, improve cardiovascular risk markers, reduce inflammation and potentially improve multiple sclerosis symptoms (36,37).

C. Prolonged periodic fasting

Fasting for 72 hours once every few months could also reap many of the benefits of a carnivorous diet. Prolonged fasting causes organs to shrink, then rejuvenate as damaged cells are eliminated and stem cell pathways are activated (38).

D. A ketogenic diet

The ketogenic diet has been well studied, with documented benefits for epilepsy, neurodegenerative diseases and autoimmune disorders. Ketones themselves are powerful anti-inflammatories (39,40).

E. Treating intestinal pathologies

If a healthy lifestyle combined with the above dietary approaches is insufficient to control your symptoms, consider working with a functional medicine practitioner familiar with gut health. If you are considering becoming a strict carnivore because you are experiencing adverse reactions to even very small amounts of plant foods, this is probably a sign of an underlying intestinal infection that should be treated.

CHAPTER 6: THE VEGETARIAN DIET

6.1. generality :

Vegetarianism is just one of a number of diets, sometimes linked to cultural reasons, beliefs or health concerns, which lead to the consumption of a variety of more or less familiar foods, in greater or lesser quantities (41).

A. Definitions :

There are many different types of diet. The most common in the human species is the omnivorous diet (42).

However, other diets are also found in human populations, such as vegetarianism, vegetarianism, frugivorism, granivorism, pescetarianism or carnivorism... Each of these diets is distinguished from the others by more or less obvious characteristics (43).

Vegetarians, also known as lacto-ovo vegetarians, eliminate meat and fish from their diet. They consume plants and animal products such as eggs and milk, but do not eat land or sea animals. They differ from vegans in that vegans eat only plants. Vegans are also known as pure vegetarians, as they also eliminate all animal products from their diet, such as eggs, cheese, milk, butter, etc. Among vegans, we can also distinguish frugivores, who eat only fruit, and crudivores, who cook food (fruit and vegetables) at no more than 48° C (44), or granivores, who eat only seeds.

Among the diets that eliminate foods of animal origin, there is one known as "vegan". Vegans are vegans (pure vegetarians, frugivores, granivores or crudivores) who, in their daily lives, in addition to meals, try not to use products that may involve the exploitation of animals. For example, these subjects are careful about the materials used in their clothing, avoid cosmetics that have been tested on animals, and do not attend shows involving animals (such as certain circus performances)... (45).

So-called pescetarians remove terrestrial meats from their diet, but still eat fish.

Some people are sometimes referred to as carnivores. This term generally applies more to animals. Indeed, to be carnivorous is to eat flesh. For humans, this term is more likely to describe a person who likes meat and uses it frequently in their diet.

It is also possible to come across people who misuse the term vegetarian. In fact, some people call themselves vegetarians because they don't eat meat for reasons of taste, even though they eat poultry - which, let's not forget, is meat - and fish. In the final analysis, these people are omnivores who eliminate certain products from their diet for a variety of reasons.

B. Reasons for vegetarianism :

Vegetarians are often not born vegetarians.
It's a lifestyle choice they acquire over time. This choice can be made for very different reasons, be they moral, medical, financial, gustatory or even psychological.

This choice to become vegetarian can be supported by several reasons for the same person (moral and health, for example).

In the case of a moral choice, it's often a question of compassion for the animal. Some people realize that if you eat an animal, it has been killed for the purpose of being eaten. These people can no longer tolerate making animals suffer in order to feed themselves, when it is possible to eat fruit and vegetables without making them suffer. So the decision is made: there will be no more meat on this person's plate. Sometimes, this decision will be more gradual, with the foods concerned being withdrawn little by little. In other words, a person who wants to become a vegetarian without abruptly changing his or her eating habits will gradually remove red meat, white meat, poultry and fish from his or her diet, depending on his or her tastes, for example.

The second reason for becoming a vegetarian is health. The vegetarian diet is seen as a model for healthy living. According to Beeson (46), using Seventh-day Adventists as an example, they live longer, healthier lives. Seventh-day Adventists have a smoke- and alcohol-free lifestyle, and their diets are very heterogeneous, including vegans, vegetarians and omnivores. We can say that they are healthy for longer, according to the same author, who explains that Seventh-day Adventists may contract a given disease at the same rate as non-Adventists, but they will survive it longer, thanks either to better access to care, a better immune system or a better lifestyle, but there is another explanation which may be that they contract the disease less. A person who is interested in his or her health, or who has health problems, may decide, in order to improve or maintain it, to select the foods he or she considers good for his or her health. This means adopting a vegetarian diet, or one very close to it. However, it's important to bear in mind that the health and longevity of Seventh-day Adventists and other communities is not due solely to the diet they follow. In fact, these people also lead healthy lifestyles, whether in terms of diet, tobacco consumption, drugs, alcohol...

Financially, a vegetarian diet can be an asset. It's expensive to feed a family with animal products at every meal. Vegetarianism helps reduce food costs. However, consumption of other food families must be increased to compensate for the absence of animal products. Further analysis of prices and quantities is needed to use finance as a reason for vegetarianism. All the more so as vegetarians, who want to lead a healthier lifestyle, will often opt for organic products. These are sometimes, but not always, more expensive than non-organic products. So it's important to weigh up the economic balance between organic and non-organic products.

Some vegetarians are simply vegetarians by choice. Indeed, a vegetarian may have removed animal products from his or her diet because they are not to his or her liking, just as an omnivore might remove vegetables from his or her diet out of aversion to them.

The vegetarian diet has a psychological component. On the one hand, a person's psychological state may encourage them to follow a path they are already on. On the other hand, the vegetarian diet can have a beneficial psychological effect on a person, as it is perceived as a positive way out of a negative period (45).

A vegetarian diet may also be chosen for religious reasons, such as Hinduism, Ladventism or Mormonism (47). In the case of a religious choice, the vegetarian diet may have been adopted from birth, and will be adopted by the whole family. But it can also be adopted during a person's life, if he or she converts to one of these religions. Some religions, which are not vegetarian, eliminate a food from their way of life, such as pork, which is eliminated among Muslims.

C. *Food consumed :*

Despite its non-use of meat, the vegetarian diet is based on a number of food families. These include: starchy foods, fruits, vegetables, legumes, pulses, oilseeds, animal products such as eggs, butter, dairy products...

Each of these foods provides different nutrients, in varying quantity and quality. A vegetarian diet is optimal when vegetarians use all these food classes in appropriate quantities.

To build a meat-free diet that best meets the body's needs, a vegetarian can rely on the vegetarian food pyramid.

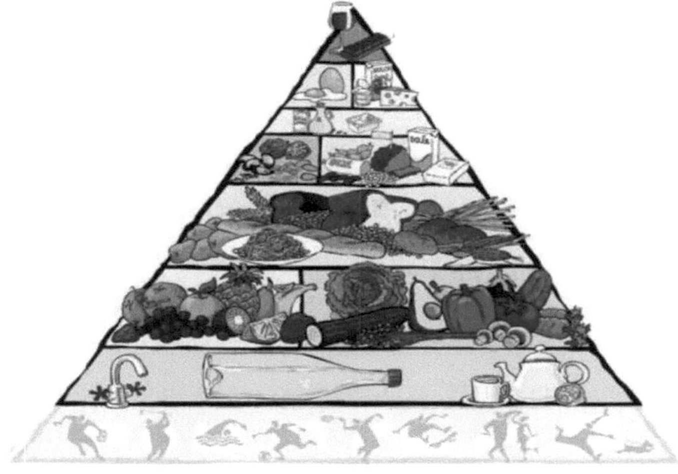

Figure 6. 1- Vegetarian food pyramid (48)

This pyramid can provide vegetarians with guidelines for a balanced diet.

At the base of this pyramid, we find the representation of physical activity. The recommendations of the French National Nutrition and Health Program (PNNS) (49) in this area apply regardless of a person's diet. For vegetarians, as for all other people, it is recommended to be physically active for at least 30 minutes a day. Added to this is at least 15 minutes' daily exposure to the sun, which is essential for vitamin D synthesis. These two activities can be carried out simultaneously.

On the upper floor, beverages must be available in abundance. These can be hot or cold. However, it is advisable to limit sugary drinks such as soft drinks. The bulk of the beverage is usually provided by water, which can be spring, mineral or tap water. But beverages such as tea, coffee (to be consumed in moderation), milk and soup also come into play. The recommended amount to drink is 2L per day (50).

Above these are fruits and vegetables. Vegetarians generally consume higher proportions of these foods than omnivores. According to the recommendations of the Agence Nationale de Sécurité Sanitaire alimentation, environnement, travail (ANSES), 4 to 6 portions of fruit and vegetables should be eaten every day (one portion corresponds to around 80g). They should be eaten at every meal, allowing for a wide variety of meals. It's best to eat seasonal fruit and vegetables, which are often of better quality and more economical.

Fruits come from plants and are, for the most part, edible, while some are poisonous or even fatal. They are rich in vitamins, in varying quantities and qualities depending on the product. Fruit is also a source of carbohydrates.

Vegetables are also derived from plants, with a generally salty taste. Of these plants, the part consumed is not always the same. Depending on the species, seeds, leaves, fruits and roots are all consumed. These vegetables are sources of carbohydrates, vitamins, proteins and trace elements.

At the top level are cereals and tubers. These foods can also be grouped under the term "starches". These products provide complex carbohydrates, also known as slow carbohydrates. They can be used as they are, like potatoes, which contain starch, or they can be used after processing, like pasta made from wheat. These processed products come in three varieties: wholemeal, semi-complete or "white", i.e. refined. In the latter case, the basic products are purified and only the inner part of the cereal is used. The husk is not retained in the final product, so the nutrients contained in the bran are eliminated. The fibers present in the husk help regulate the immune response, while phenolic acids, among other phytochemicals, have antioxidant activity. These effects are greatly diminished or even virtually eliminated when wheat is refined (51). Starchy foods should be included at every meal, as they make a major contribution to energy intake. This food family is therefore necessary for daily activity, but not sufficient.

At the top of the range are protein products. These include legumes, pulses and by-products such as soya milk. They should be consumed daily, with 1 to 2 portions per day for legumes and 50 to 150 g for protein foods.

Legumes form fruits that are pods and are used as vegetables. In fact, both legume fruits and vegetables are often referred to as vegetables.

Dried vegetables, on the other hand, are legume seeds that are also edible and sometimes assimilated to vegetables.

These legumes and pulses, assimilated to vegetables, are also sources of carbohydrates, vitamins, proteins and trace elements in varying quantities.

On the same level of the vegetarian food pyramid are oleaginous fruits. They are a source of lipids and should be consumed at a daily rate of 30-60g.

Vegetable oils and fats, also sources of lipids, provide the human body with essential fatty acids and Iiposoluble vitamins. The recommended daily amount is 2 to 4 tablespoons for an adult.

If we continue to climb the food pyramid, we find eggs and dairy products on the same floor. These foods are all of animal origin, and therefore all sources of animal protein. Dairy products are also sources of calcium and various vitamins. They should be consumed regularly, with a daily intake of around 250 g of milk. Dairy products can be found in the form of butter, cream, milk, cheese and yoghurt... However, when milk is in the form of cheese, it should be consumed in moderation, due to the concentrated fat content of this type of food.

At the top of the pyramid are alcohol and sweets. These products are not necessary for the body. They can be used for personal satisfaction and pleasure, in reasonable quantities.

6.2. Health benefits of vegetarianism :

The vegetarian diet, as we saw earlier, removes a number of products from a person's diet. As a result, the nutrient intakes provided by a vegetarian diet are quite different from those provided by an omnivorous diet. These differences in intake give rise to more or less direct health benefits for the vegetarian.

A. Weight and obesity :

Today, overweight and obesity are a public health problem.

All health professionals are working together to find a solution to this scourge, which is growing by the day. The reasons for these weight problems are varied: an increase in the number of meals eaten "on the run", poor eating habits, a more sedentary lifestyle...

The assessment of a person's excess body fat is based not only on their weight, but also on their Body Mass Index (BMI). This BMI is not directly applicable to growing children, or to people of the 3rd age, so standards need to be adjusted for these types of people (52). For example, in children, staturo-ponderal curves, which are a visual adaptation of BMI standards, should be used to detect potential overweight as early as possible. Similarly, in the case of a senior citizen, it's important to take into account the decrease in height, due in particular to osteoporosis. BMI corresponds to weight in kilograms divided by height in meters squared.

B. *Vegetarianism-obesity relationship :*

Vegetarians tend to have lower daily calorie intakes than non-vegetarians. In fact, vegetarians consume an average of 2070 kcal per day, compared with an average of 2120 kcal for omnivores (53,54). In effect, the quantity of meat removed from the diet by vegetarians is replaced by foods with a lower caloric content for the same volume.

Vegetarians have a lower body mass index than omnivores (55), which could be due to a higher intake of fiber and a lower intake of animal fats. For example, a meta-analysis (56) shows that the average BMI of a non-vegetarian is 28.26, whereas for a vegetarian, the average BMI is 25.48. As a result, their weight is closer than that of non-vegetarians to the ideal weight that a person should have according to various parameters: sex, age, height... The ideal weight is used to determine whether a person is overweight or underweight (57). This ideal weight can be calculated using a variety of methods:

- Lorentz formula (58) :

Ideal weight = height (cm) -100 - ((height (cm) - 150) /n)

n = 4 for a man and 2.5 for a woman

- Devine's formula (59):

Ideal weight for a man = 45.4 + 0.89 × (height (cm) - 152.4) + 0.45

Ideal weight for a woman = 45.4 + 0.89 × (height (cm) - 152.4) These formulas only apply to people over 18.

l.Diabetes :

According to the World Health Organization (WHO) (60), diabetes is characterized by higher-than-normal blood sugar levels, which occur when the pancreas doesn't produce enough insulin, or when the body doesn't know how to use this hormone properly. It is diagnosed when there are two fasting blood glucose readings above 1.26g/L (7mmol/L), or one blood glucose reading above 2g/L (11.1mmol/L), regardless of the time of sampling. Diabetes can lead to serious complications, particularly of the nerves and blood vessels.

There are several types of diabetes. The two main types are: type 1 diabetes, known as insulin-dependent diabetes, and type 2 diabetes, also known as non-insulin-dependent diabetes. These two types of diabetes have very different pathophysiological mechanisms, and therefore require different treatments.

Insulin-dependent diabetes is often discovered in childhood, and results from a lack of insulin production by the body. Treatment of type 1 diabetes therefore requires insulin injections.

Non-insulin-dependent diabetes is most often found in older patients. It is also known as fatty diabetes, and depends in part on the patient's diet. Type 2 diabetes results from increased resistance to insulin receptors. As a result, blood sugar levels are not regulated as required. The treatment of this type of diabetes involves various therapeutic classes: biguanides, hypoglycemic sulfonamides, glinides, glitazones, α-glucosidase inhibitors, incretinomimetics... Insulin is not prescribed as a first-line treatment. Because of the dietary component, the first line of treatment in the discovery of type 2 diabetes is to implement hygienic-dietary measures. After 3 to 6 months, if these measures fail, they should not be abandoned, but drug treatment should be added, using one or more of the pharmacological classes listed above. Subsequently, after several years of treatment, type 2 diabetes may become insulin-requiring. Patients suffering from non-insulin-dependent diabetes will then warrant additional insulin injections.

As we said earlier, nutrition is an important factor for type 2 diabetics. A type 2 diabetic patient must have a protein intake corresponding to 15% of his or her total energy intake. These proteins must be provided in equivalent quantities by animal and vegetable products. These patients often consume large quantities of meat and fish. Their treatment must therefore begin with a reduction in these meat intakes. In fact, animal proteins can be provided by other products, such as dairy products and eggs.

Diabetes is not the only pathology influenced by a person's diet - there are many others. Diet also plays a part in the group of pathologies known as cardiovascular diseases.

C. *Cardiovascular diseases* :

Cardiovascular disease is the leading cause of death worldwide, according to the WHO. Several studies show that the mortality rate from coronary heart disease is lower in vegetarians than in non-vegetarians (61). Indeed, Key et al (62) report that the mortality rate from ischemic heart disease is lower in vegetarians than in omnivores. Similarly, studies by Battaglia et al. (63) and Huang et al. (64) concur.

This lower mortality rate from coronary heart disease s is due to the fact that vegetarians have lower cholesterol levels and a lower BMI s.

According to the WHO, cardiovascular pathologies include various disorders of the heart and blood vessels, which are classified into different sub-categories:

- hypertension,

- coronary heart disease,

- cerebrovascular diseases,

- peripheral arterial disease,

- heart failure,

- rheumatic heart disease,

- congenital heart disease,

- cardiomyopathies,

- deep vein thrombosis and pulmonary embolism.

All these pathologies require different treatments, as well as a variety of follow-up therapies.

Risk factors for some of these pathologies are numerous. Rheumatic heart disease and congenital heart disease are genetic in origin, and the risk factors dependent on the individual are fewer. Risk factors for other cardiovascular diseases include gender, age, personal and family history, weight, smoking, diet, physical inactivity, stress and type 2 diabetes. Some of these can be influenced (weight, smoking, nutrition, sedentary lifestyle, type 2 diabetes), others cannot (age, sex, history).

Several studies show that blood cholesterol levels are lower in vegetarians than in non-vegetarians (65). In fact, cholesterol levels are 0.61 mmol/L lower in vegetarians than in non-vegetarians. A patient suffers from dyslipidemia when his or her total cholesterol level in the blood is above 5.20 mmol/L, or 2.0 g/L, or his or her LDL cholesterol (Low Density Lipoprotein) level in the blood is above 4.1 mmol/L, or 1.6 g/L.

In Table 4, we can see that HDL-cholesterol (High Density Protein) levels are virtually identical regardless of the type of diet followed. However, LDL-cholesterol levels are 0.43 mmol/L lower in vegetarians than in omnivores, which is reflected in total cholesterol levels. Statistical tests demonstrate the heterogeneity of the study subjects.

In addition, a study by De Biase et al (65) shows that the vegetarian diet is associated with lower levels of triglycerides, total cholesterol and LDL-cholesterol than the omnivorous diet. fl also appears that phytochemicals, found in greater quantities in the vegetarian diet than in the omnivorous diet, exert an influence on cholesterol levels, via various mechanisms (66).

We can therefore see that omnivorous subjects are more prone to dyslipidemia than vegetarians, but also than other types of diet (vegans, and pescetarians).

The first step in treating dyslipidemia is to adopt hygienic-dietary measures, in particular by reducing lipid intake and improving it by consuming mainly vegetable fats and favoring polyunsaturated fatty acids.

If these hygienic and dietary measures are not sufficient, Statins or fibrates can be used to treat the condition.

As far as hypertension is concerned, the vegetarian diet can bring significant benefits, with its lower salt intake compared to an omnivorous diet (63), and a lower incidence of obesity, as we saw earlier. A vegetarian subject takes his or her entire lifestyle into account, and thus tends towards a healthier lifestyle. In fact, the percentage of vegetarians who regularly drink alcohol is lower than that of non-vegetarians, and vegetarians smoke less (67). All these factors can lead to a reduction of 2 to 10 mmHg in systolic or diastolic blood pressure (61).

In these hygienic-dietary measures, we do not observe any reduction in meat or fish consumption, apart from controlling the origin of lipids. However, the significant reduction in blood pressure in vegetarians compared with non-vegetarians leads us to believe that a vegetarian diet may contribute to reducing the incidence of hypertension (61).

As a second-line treatment, if dietary and hygienic measures are not sufficient, medication may be used. However, dietary measures implemented in the first instance should not be discarded.

Other cardiovascular diseases all share the same risk factors. What's more, they can be complications of dyslipidemia or hypertension, which is why it's so important to manage these conditions properly.

In the vegetarian population, the reduction in the risk of death from stroke is small but present. Once again, the vegetarian diet can act on the risk factors for this pathology (61). Indeed, increased consumption of fruit and vegetables is one of the many factors contributing to the decline in the number of strokes in Europe and North America (68). Let's not forget that this increase in vegetable consumption is a feature of the vegetarian diet. Similarly, we saw earlier that a vegetarian diet contributes to a reduction in total cholesterol and blood pressure, which are themselves factors reducing the risk of stroke (69).

The vegetarian diet can therefore be proposed as a regulator of the various risk factors for cardiovascular disease. These different pathologies may in fact be linked to each other. Acting on one pathology also acts on the others. For example, a vegetarian diet can make a person healthier than a non-vegetarian. What's more, a vegetarian diet on a larger scale could reduce the mortality rate from cardiovascular pathologies.

As we've seen, the vegetarian diet can have an effect on a number of cardiovascular pathologies, but it's not the only one. Thanks to its absence of animal proteins, the vegetarian diet can also facilitate kidney function.

D. *Chronic renal failure:*

The kidneys are the body's organs of elimination and detoxification. They are sensitive and can be affected by many factors: diet, tobacco, alcohol, medication...

The kidneys have four main functions: elimination of nitrogenous waste products, maintenance of internal composition, control of blood pressure, endocrine function of the kidney.

Renal function is assessed by monitoring glomerular filtration rate (GFR). Several biological parameters can be used to check this GFR. These include creatinine, creatinine clearance (calculated according to the Cockcroft and Gault formula or the MDRD (Modification of Diet in Renal Disease) method), measurement of renal clearance of a substance, and inulin clearance. Depending on the GFR result, there are different stages of renal disease.

The first action to be taken in renal failure is the prevention and management of risk factors. These risk factors are :

- diabetes, which needs to be carefully controlled;

- arterial hypertension, which must be treated with medication in addition to hygienic and dietary measures;

- dyslipidemia.

Anemia, vitamin D deficiency and phosphocalcium disorders should be corrected.

It should be borne in mind that the vegetarian diet may decrease creatinine production (70). This decrease in creatinine production reduces creatinine clearance and may therefore lead to an error in the assessment of DF
G .

However, a study by Barsotti et al (71) showed a significant improvement in creatinine clearance, and hence renal function, in patients with renal failure after switching from an omnivorous to a vegetarian diet.

Thus, even if a vegetarian diet does not directly benefit renal function (72), it can act on the risk factors of chronic renal failure. By acting on these risk factors, it slows down the irreversible deterioration of renal function in chronic renal failure.

E. Oncology :

Cancers are many and varied. They correspond to the development of tumor cells in the body, in a specific site. There are two types of tumor: benign and malignant. The aggressiveness of a tumor is assessed according to its capacity to develop metastases, i.e. tumor foci at a distance from the primary tumor.

For a tumor to develop, at least 5 or 6 mutations must occur. Age is therefore a risk factor for cancer. But it's not the only risk factor. Sex, smoking, alcohol, sexual behavior, environment, personal and family history are all factors that can lead to the development of cancer. Each risk factor is of greater or lesser importance, depending on the type of cancer in question.

Several studies have been carried out on the link between cancer and vegetarianism, providing contradictory information (64). It appears that, taking all cancers together, the incidence of cancer is lower in vegetarians than in non-vegetarians (73).

One study found a direct link between red meat consumption and the incidence of colon cancer (74). Accordingly, the study by Battaglia Richi et al. estimated that 10% of cases of colon cancer could be avoided if processed meat consumption were totally abandoned (63).

Similarly, the risk of intestinal cancer increases with regular consumption of more than 500g of red meat per week (63).

Prostate cancer incidence is also significantly higher in non-vegetarians (75).

Red meat is recognized as a significant contributor to the increased risk of esophageal cancer, while fish consumption of around 50 g per day brings a 38% reduction in the risk of the same cancer (76). This protection against cancer by fish is thought to be due to the presence in its tissues of a high level of omega-3 fatty acids, which may have anti-carcinogenic properties (75).

Although the vegetarian diet seems to have a beneficial impact on the incidence of various cancers, it seems possible that this is not only due to the absence of meat in the diet, but also probably due to the increased consumption of fruit, vegetables, seeds and various nuts, which would provide the body with protective elements against cancers (75).

However, the vegetarian diet can also have its drawbacks, both in terms of physical and moral health. So if we want to adopt a vegetarian diet, we need to think carefully about how we go about it.

F. Food-borne diseases :

Food can also be the cause of the transmission of multiple diseases, whose pathogens can be viruses, bacteria or parasites, but also toxic chemicals or toxins (77). These pathologies vary in severity, and can even be fatal.

One such pathology is salmonellosis. This is a bacterial infection caused by Salmonella enterobacteria (78). Salmonellosis can cause fever, diarrhea, vomiting and abdominal pain. In some cases, this infection can be fatal. The main sources of Salmonella contamination are meat (particularly poultry), fish products, eggs and dairy products (79).

In the category of viruses, we can take hepatitis A as an example. This virus is transmitted by the hands, or by contaminated food. The main culprits are drinking water, undercooked shellfish, fruit and raw vegetables (80). The major signs of hepatitis A infection are fever, severe asthenia, nausea accompanied by abdominal pain, followed by jaundice and sometimes pruritus (81).

Parasites can also be found in human food (82). For example, undercooked beef can be the source of Taenia saginata contamination. The consumption of undercooked pork, on the other hand, can result in the transmission of Taenia solium. Colonization by T. saginata is asymptomatic in humans (83), and has no major consequences for the human organism, whereas T. solium can cause human cysticercosis, which can be fatal. Infection with T. solium, more commonly known as tapeworm, causes symptoms such as abdominal pain, nausea, diarrhea or constipation (84). When the worm reaches maturity, infection may be asymptomatic for several years. Subsequently, the larvae can develop in muscles, skin, eyes and the central nervous system, forming cysts. When cysts form in the brain, the pathology is called neurocysticercosis. Cysts can cause severe headaches, blindness, convulsions and sometimes epileptic seizures, leading to death (85).

Creutzfeldt-Jakob disease (CJD), another fatal pathology, can be contracted by eating infected beef (86). Infection with CJD occurs via the mutated prion protein, a very small infectious agent (87). The disease causes dementia, myoclonus and cerebellar syndromes (88). It is rapidly progressive, and always fatal (89).

Food can also be a source of heavy metal poisoning. Take mercury, for example. Mercury poisoning has many different origins, but among them, the body can be poisoned by eating fish whose flesh is loaded with mercury (90). This type of intoxication is the cause of various disorders of the central and peripheral nervous systems. Thus, in a subject suffering from mercury intoxication, we can observe ataxia, tremors, instability when walking, and hypoesthesia (91). There are various sources of mercury, which may be natural and/or anthropogenic (92). Once emitted, mercury contaminates a link in the food chain, accumulating until it reaches the last link in the chain (93).

A vegetarian diet cannot completely avoid this type of poisoning, but it can limit it.

Not all diseases that can be transmitted by animal products are completely excluded, since some can also be transmitted by plants. But a vegetarian diet helps to reduce the prevalence of these diseases.

To conclude on the benefits of vegetarianism, we can see that vegetarianism has positive effects on health. For example, it reduces the prevalence of a number of pathologies. Of course, this type of diet does not eliminate all the risks of pathologies, whether chronic or acute, that we have just explored.

6.3 Disadvantages of vegetarianism :

Vegetarianism is therefore a healthy way of eating, with positive health benefits for the vegetarian. However, vegetarianism can also have negative effects on health, notably deficiencies. Indeed, vegetarianism can give rise to various deficiencies. What's more, vegetarianism may not be suitable for everyone. So let's take a look at the disadvantages inherent in a vegetarian diet, focusing first on iron.

A. Iron status :

Iron is a very important micronutrient in human nutrition. It performs a variety of functions in the body. In particular, it is the central molecule of hemoglobin, but it is also found in myoglobin for oxygen transport, and is involved in many other mechanisms.

The body's iron requirements are different for men, women, children and the elderly. Intake must therefore be adapted to the individual's profile. For example, a man needs to absorb 1 mg of iron per day, compared with 1.5 mg for a woman, while a pregnant woman may need to absorb up to 5 mg per day. In order to meet these requirements, an adequate intake of iron from the diet is necessary: 8 mg per day for men, 18 mg for women, and up to 27 mg for pregnant women. Iron deficiency occurs when iron absorption falls short of the body's needs.

Iron deficiency has various physical, mental, physiological and behavioral consequences for the body (94).

Iron is supplied by different foods and in different forms. Haem iron is provided by meat, while non-haem iron is provided by plants. Heme iron is better absorbed by the body than non-heme iron (95), which is why we believe that vegetarians are more at risk of iron deficiency than omnivores.

In addition, various substances such as phytates, which are also present in plants, chelate iron and are therefore responsible for a reduction in the bioavailability of iron from the alimentary bolus (94,96).

However, we can also see that the simultaneous intake of iron-containing foods and foods containing ascorbic acid increases the body's bioavailability of non-heme iron (97), mainly due to ascorbic acid's ability to convert ferric iron into ferrous iron.

We can see that meat provides 15% of the iron intake of an omnivore, i.e. as much as vegetables, and most of the iron provided to omnivores comes from cereals. Similarly, the majority of a vegetarian's iron intake comes from cereals, closely followed by plants. In fact, when a vegetarian eliminates meat from his or her diet, he or she also increases his or her intake of vegetables and pulses, fruit and, in most cases, wholegrain cereals (96). What's more, for both omnivores and vegetarians, we observe that 15% of the iron acquired comes from breakfast cereals.

B. Fat intake :

Previously, I highlighted the fact that vegetarians have a lower lipid intake than omnivores. This lower lipid content in the diet is responsible for a reduced risk of developing cardiovascular disease. However, it may also be at the root of a low intake of essential fatty acids.

Certain omega-3 and omega-6 unsaturated fatty acids (FAs) are known as essential fatty acids, as they must be supplied by the diet. Only linolenic acid (ALA) and linoleic acid (LA) are truly essential to the human organism, as they cannot be biosynthesized in sufficient quantities by the body (97).

The other essential fatty acids, eicosapentaenoic acid (EP A), docosahexaenoic acidB(DHA), linolenic acid, dihomo-y-linolenic acid and arachidonic acid, can be synthesized from ALA and LA . The biosynthesis of these polyunsaturated fatty acids involves the same enzymes. So, when omega-3 deficiency is perceived, omega-6 biosynthesis is increased. This compensation in biosynthesis does not avoid the harmful effects of omega 3 deficiency, but it does maintain the total level of polyunsaturated fatty acids, thus ensuring the membrane stability of the body's cells (98).

Fatty acids play different roles in the body, with omega 3 and omega 6 playing opposite roles. In fact, they are metabolized into various molecules involved in coagulation, regulation of blood LDL cholesterol and blood sugar levels, and regulation of the inflammatory and immune response (99).

In fact, omega-3 fatty acids are essential for the construction and proper functioning of the brain (100).

An excess of omega 3, on the other hand, can lead to coagulation problems, high LDL cholesterol levels, low blood sugar levels and a weak immune and inflammatory response. In fact, if omega-3 intake is too high, its metabolism will be too, and consequently the activity of its metabolites will be increased.

In contrast, a deficiency in omega-3 could lead to a rise in blood sugar levels, or an overly strong immune or inflammatory response. fl is therefore in every human being's interest to have a balanced intake of omega-3 and omega-6 fats, in line with the body's needs. It is therefore recommended that the omega 6 / omega 3 ratio should be close to 5 for adults (101).

Omega 3 can be found mainly in fish for those on an omnivorous or pescetarian diet. Vegetarians, on the other hand, will have to rely on other foods to meet their omega-3 needs. Flaxseed is rich in omega-3. Take herring, for example, which has an omega-3 content of 3g per 100g (102). fl is in fact less rich in omega-3s than flaxseed, which provides over 16g of omega-3s per 100g of seed (103). However, the body is not designed to digest whole flaxseed properly, and so cannot absorb the omega-3 fatty acids it contains, so fl ground flaxseed should be used to optimize absorption, fl fl flaxseed oil can also be used. Other vegetable sources of omega-3 fatty acids are also available. Chia seeds, walnuts and walnut oil all contain them. For vegetarians, pulses also provide omega-3. The ratio of omega 3 to omega 6 varies from one vegetable oil to another, which is why it's a good idea to consume oils from different origins to vary your intake. The compositions of other oils rich in omega-3 fatty acids are listed in Appendix 2. For example, purslane oil stands out from other oils with an omega-3 fatty acid content of 32.4% (190). But purslane is not only consumed in oil form. Purslane, Portulaca olerácea L., is a plant that can also be used raw or cooked. Not only does this plant offer interesting nutritional properties (104), it is also used as a medicinal plant.

As for vegetables, a food family consumed in large quantities by vegetarians, they are a poor source of omega-3 FAs. Similarly, dairy products are not a major source of omega-3 fatty acids. In fact, cow's milk has an omega-3 content of 1.4g per 100g.

C. Other nutrients :

There are many other nutrients we need in our diet. Among them, several are the subject of debate concerning their intake in the vegetarian diet. For example, the intake of vitamins B12 and D, as well as calcium, is a bone of contention.

Vitamin B12 deficiency is at the root of a variety of manifestations: hematological, neuropsychiatric, epithelial, vascular; indeed, vitamin B12 is a ubiquitous coenzyme involved in reactions leading to DNA (Deoxyribonucleic Acid) synthesis. Vitamin B12 deficiency therefore alters DNA synthesis, which is at the root of these various syndromes.

The human body requires a vitamin B12 intake of 3 µg/day [105]. As we can see from Table 8, only animal products contain vitamin B12. Therefore, it is legitimate to think that vegetarians may be deficient in vitamin B12. However, we can see that eggs (an animal product) are a source of this vitamin. Similarly, cow's milk provides 45 µg of vitamin B12 per 100 ml. So a person following a vegetarian diet and consuming dairy products regularly should not suffer from vitamin B12 deficiency. A study by Elmadfa and Singer shows that serum vitamin B12 levels are lower in vegetarians than in omnivores, but vegetarians are not necessarily deficient (106). Although vegetarians have lower plasma vitamin B12 levels than omnivores, these levels are not low enough to indicate deficiency.

Vitamin D deficiency can lead to a variety of disorders, the main one being osteoporosis, but also osteomalacia, sarcopenia, reduced muscular performance and proprioceptivity, and impaired cognitive function (107). The recommended intake of vitamin D is 800 to 1000 IU per day (108). Available sources of vitamin D are exposure to UVB (Ultra-Violet type B) sunlight and, in the diet, mainly oily fish. On the dietary side, egg yolks, mushrooms and dairy products are low sources of vitamin D.

It should be noted that the vitamin D produced by the skin during exposure to the sun, as well as that found in oily fish, is vitamin D3. Whereas that found in plants is vitamin D2. Vitamin D2 is less effective in maintaining adequate circulating vitamin D levels, as its half-life is shorter than that of vitamin D3 [109], and it is also less stable than vitamin D3 [110]. This difference between vitamin D2 and vitamin D3 may explain why vegetarians are more at risk of vitamin D deficiency than omnivores.

However, vitamin D deficiency is common in France. In a study by Vemay et al [111], 80% of the population studied was more or less severely deficient in vitamin D. The characteristics of the population studied did not assess the type of diet consumed. Thus, we can see that vitamin D deficiency is common in France, regardless of the type of diet consumed. Epidemiological studies of this deficiency are few and far between. It is therefore difficult to incriminate vegetarianism as the main cause of vitamin D deficiency.

Calcium is one of the main nutrients required for healthy bones. According to ANSES, the recommended daily calcium intake for adults is 900 mg (112). Calcium seems to be less well absorbed by a person eating a vegetarian diet than by a person eating an omnivorous diet (110,111). This suggests that vegetarian consumers may be at greater risk of low bone mineral density and fracture (113). However, it would appear that the calcium requirements of vegetarians are lower than those of omnivores (114). Furthermore, it appears that the bone mineral density of vegetarians and non-vegetarians is similar (115), and the fracture rate is similar between the two groups, so the vegetarian diet is able to support bone health in the human body (113).

D. *Vegetarianism in pregnancy and infancy:*

It is important to assess the impact of a vegetarian diet on infants, children and teenagers, as well as the impact of a vegetarian diet on women during pregnancy and when breastfeeding their babies. The vegetarian diet, often seen as the cause of various nutritional deficiencies, could in fact be responsible for growth disorders.

During pregnancy, a woman's nutritional requirements change. For example, a pregnant woman will require an energy intake of 2200 to 2900 kcal per day on average, compared with 1900 to 2500 kcal per day for a non-pregnant woman (116). However, the fact that a vegetarian woman can have a successful pregnancy without negative effects for herself or her baby is well documented.

(117) . As long as the vegetarian diet is well planned, it can meet the particular nutritional needs of pregnancy (118).

The vegetarian diet results in a lower calorie intake, and a deficit in animal proteins, vitamins D and B12, and iron too. However, children's growth and development are not affected by these low intakes. In fact, we can see that, despite the low calorie intake of the vegetarian diet, energy intake is sufficient to ensure proper development compared to a non-vegetarian child.

(118) .

However, it is important to remember that infants under 1 year of age cannot be fed vegetable drinks (119). These plant-based beverages do not contain the nutrients required to cover an infant's needs. If a child is not breast-fed, and we do not wish to give him or her a formula containing lactose, we can use lactose-free infant formulas and follow-on formulas, or formulas based on vegetable proteins.

During lactation, milk from a vegetarian mother seems to differ significantly from that of an omnivorous mother in its composition. This is because milk reflects the characteristics of the mother's diet. Thus, the milk of a vegetarian woman will be less concentrated in long-chain saturated fatty acids, and have a higher content of polyunsaturated fatty acids than that of an omnivorous woman (117). As a result, there have been a few cases of growth difficulties in children fed by vegetarian mothers, but despite this, vegetarian women can still successfully breastfeed their children. In fact, despite some differences in fatty acid content, the milk of a vegetarian woman is very similar to that of a non-vegetarian woman in terms of minerals, trace elements, lactose and total fatty acids (120), but is less concentrated in vitamin B12(121).

What's more, we can see that milk produced by a vegetarian woman is lower in environmental contaminants and additives (120). This means healthier milk for the child.

After that, we need to be vigilant and aware that the diet must be adapted to the age and type of person, and possibly to pathologies. A diet that may be suitable for an adult will not necessarily be suitable for a child (120).

After breast-feeding, if this has taken place, or after the child has reached 6 months of age, comes the stage of dietary diversification. At this stage, the child is very fragile from a nutritional point of view, and may require vitamin D and iron supplements (120). Other deficiencies may also be observed, such as deficiencies in calories, protein, vitamin B12, calcium, zinc, phosphorus and iron. Children of this age need to be carefully monitored. They are vulnerable and need to be supplemented if necessary.

Growth in children aged 18 months to 5 years is significantly impaired, probably due to the lower caloric intake of a vegetarian diet compared with an omnivorous diet. Thus, vegetarian children have shorter stature and lower weight than omnivorous children at the same ages (120).

For children aged 5 to 11, the possible problem lies in the habits they will develop. In fact, these eating habits developed in childhood will continue into adulthood. It is therefore necessary to provide the vegetarian child with the good eating habits of his diet, so that he retains them in adulthood, and his body does not suffer from an avoidable deficiency (120).

In adolescence, the hematocrit and hemoglobin values of vegetarians are found to be within the norms, but also similar to those of omnivorous adolescents. However, a zinc deficiency may have set in. The zinc provided by plants is often chelated by the phytic acids found in unrefined cereals. This chelation results in products with low solubility, so zinc absorption is reduced (122).

Vegetarianism in adolescence is also often assimilated and/or associated with an eating disorder, which can lead to menstrual disorders. If an eating disorder is present, it should be treated. But a vegetarian diet is not always an eating disorder.

What's more, adolescents undergo considerable physiological stress, which can accentuate the deficiencies that can be caused by a vegetarian diet (123). It is therefore important to be vigilant regarding the various nutritional intakes required, and supplementation may be necessary.

We can see that a vegetarian diet can be adopted at any age. However, some nutrients need to be monitored to avoid deficiencies, and appropriate supplements may need to be taken to make up for any shortfalls. A vegetarian diet in children may even be beneficial for cardiovascular, degenerative and metabolic diseases in adults (120).

E) Vegetarianism for seniors :

An elderly person, also known as a senior citizen, is defined as being over the age of 65. However, this limit should be treated with caution and adapted according to the individual's state of health. In fact, a person under 65 may be considered elderly if he or she is taking a lot of medication every day (more than 5 a day), or if he or she is bedridden, disabled or unable to look after himself or herself. Likewise, a 70-year-old with no health problems and full physical and mental capacity should not be considered elderly.

The senior vegetarian is a rare and little-known patient. However, it's important to take an interest in them, to provide them with the best possible support in their approach and their health.

The elderly omnivore can suffer from a number of pathologies (124): hypertension and other cardiovascular diseases, type 2 diabetes, degenerative diseases, osteoporosis... As we have already seen, vegetarianism can be an asset in the face of some of these, but for other pathologies the situation is different.

Elderly people have many reasons for being vegetarians. The same reasons apply as for younger subjects: compassion for animals, health reasons, psychological reasons. But seniors may also have been vegetarians for many years and not wish to change their diet. For others, it's the act of eating itself. Over time, a distaste for certain foods, particularly meat, may develop. Oral pathologies may also be responsible for a change in the senior's eating habits: loss of teeth, chewing and swallowing difficulties(125) ...

The risks of these oral pathologies are to reduce the intake in quantity and quality of the various nutrients required by the body, and thus lead to undernutrition from which it is difficult to extricate the subject, f l it is therefore important to support the elderly subject so that he or she does not suffer from undernutrition, whether vegetarian or not.

Thus, an elderly person who becomes malnourished easily suffers from sarcopenia, excess weight and fat mass, and has a lower total energy expenditure and lower resting energy expenditure than a younger person. Protein metabolism is also impaired. Elderly patients are often less physically active than younger subjects (124). The elderly patient is therefore a fragile subject, and it is essential that his or her diet be adapted to avoid causing him or her harm (125).

CHAPTER 7: THE OMNIVOROUS DIET

7.1 Introduction

Like monkeys and bears, humans have an omnivorous diet, which means they eat a variety of foods:

S Of animal origin: such as meat, fish, milk and its derivatives, eggs...

S Of plant origin: such as bread, fruit, vegetables...

To be able to process all these varied foods, omnivorous animals have adaptive anatomical structures in their craniums and digestive tracts.

7.2. Observation of the cranial cavity in humans

A. *Observation of the cranial cavity in humans*

- The human skull is made up of two jaws, an upper and a lower.

- A number of different teeth are attached to each jaw.

- The lower jaw has both vertical and lateral movements.

- The lower jaw can make these movements thanks to the masticatory muscles, or facial muscles, strong muscles that can be felt by touching the face when chewing.

B. *Human dentition*

1. Tooth structure

The tooth is a predominantly mineralized organ found on both jaws, used for chewing food.

Each tooth is made up of two parts:

-The crown: the visible part of the tooth.

- The root: is the invisible part of the tooth that sinks into the gum and is attached to the jawbone. The number of roots for each tooth varies according to its type (incisors and canines have a single root, premolars have one or two roots, and molars have either two or three roots).

2. types of teeth: shape and role

Adult man has four types of teeth, all different in shape and function.

- Incisors: are the teeth on the front of each jaw, have a single root and are sharp like a knife; their role is to cut food.

- Canines: next to the incisors, they have a single root and are pointed. Their role is to shred food, especially meat.

- Premolars: located between canines and molars, they have one or two roots and a flattened surface. Their role is to crush food.

- The last type of tooth, the molars, are found on the inside of the mouth. They have two or three roots, a flattened surface and their role is to crush food.

Man is said to have a complete set of teeth.

3. Dental formula

The dental formula is a mathematical expression that represents the number of each type of tooth in half a jaw.

The dental formula is expressed as a fraction, with the teeth of the upper half jaw in the numerator and the teeth of the lower half jaw in the denominator.

We note the number of teeth followed by the first letter, for example: 31+ 1C+ 3PM + 3M (I for incisor, C for canine, PM for premolar, and M for molar).

4) Observation of lower jaw movements

The lower jaw articulates with the skull at the level of the articulating condyle.

The articulating condyle has a rounded shape that allows the lower jaw to move vertically and laterally.

7.3. Human digestive tract organs
A.The journey of food through the digestive tract

After mastication, the next process is deglutination: the food bolus passes through the digestive tract in the following order:

Mouth-esophagus-stomach-small intestine-large intestine-rectum-anus

7.4. Human adaptation to an omnivorous diet
Man is said to be adapted to his omnivorous diet because *the structures and organs* he has are perfectly suited to processing foods of animal and plant origin (you'll have this course in detail in 3rd year college), here are a few examples:

- It has a complete dentition, with a variety of teeth in response to different foods.
- Molars for shredding meat
- Molars with a flattened surface for crushing food, especially vegetable food.

- The lower jaw performs different vertical and lateral movements.
- The cranium has very strong masticatory muscles.

The omnivore diet is the **most recommended diet for good health!** From the Latin *omni* (everything) and *vorare* (to eat), an omnivorous diet means eating all kinds of foods (vegetables, fruit, meat, fish, dairy products, cereals, etc.), depending on the season and taste. Human beings are omnivores by nature, their digestive organs enabling them to digest both plant and animal foods.

CONCLUSION

In nature, living beings are in balance, each feeding in their own way: some are producers, others consumers, super consumers, predators, super predators and even decomposers, in order to maintain health and promote growth.

Since our earliest origins, millions of years ago, human digestive physiology has enabled us to digest and assimilate all types of natural foods, making us highly adaptable to environmental changes. However, the ratio of animal to vegetable intake has slowly evolved over time towards an increasingly camel-like tendency, and the earliest tools used by early *homo* ancestors were designed for butchering carcasses and crushing bones.

Early man was distinguished by his search for quality, nutrient-rich foods, which helped develop his brain. Low-carbohydrate, low-calorie plant foods were not enough. The consumption of bone marrow certainly contributed to brain growth, as did wild game rich in omega 3 and low in saturated fats, and shellfish and fish rich in omega 3.

Meat provides glucose through gluconeogenesis in times of drought and lack of vegetation, and helps maintain a regular food supply whatever the climate. The emergence of the human species could be the result of the selection of omnivorous individuals having acquired a regular supply of foodstuffs of high nutritional value.

With *homo georgiens* 1.7 million years ago, the hunting character of our ancestors becomes clear, and their attraction for game is such that they leave Africa to venture into colder climates, abandoning the tropics and their luxuriant vegetation for good game fed on green grass...

Its gracile jaw, like that of homo sapiens, shows that it already eats less tough vegetation, which it has replaced with meat.

With *homo erectus*, the consumption of herbivorous animals became even more important, with social organization based on the hunting of big game. Cooking foodstuffs, particularly plants (including starches), would also have favored encephalization by releasing plant nutrients.

It allows more calories to be absorbed more quickly, and man spends less time feeding and chewing, his dentition decreasing sharply from this point onwards. *Homo erectus* emigrated far from Africa, adapting to all climates thanks to an omnivorous diet with a strong tendency towards meat. A frugivorous vegan hominid would not have been able to survive in the north, and would not have felt the need to move far from the tropics.

Homo sapiens, i.e. modern man, is not the descendant of a branch of *&homo erectus* that emigrated north hundreds of thousands of years ago, and disappeared. *Homo sapiens* appeared in Africa from *&homo* left behind around 200,000 years ago, and stayed there until around 60,000 years ago, when some of them began to spread across the globe. Today's Africans are those who did not emigrate and have remained adapted to the lifestyle of our common ancestors. *Homo sapiens* arrived in Europe at the height of the Ice Age around 40,000 years ago. Despite this major environmental change, they adapted well. The hunter-gatherer Cro-magnons of the Dordogne could consume more than a kilo of meat a day, but frequent periods of fasting linked to an uncertain supply and intense physical activity in the cold enabled them to burn and autolyze the toxins generated by the digestive metabolism of meat.

In fact, it seems that they never exceeded 50% meat in their diet, despite their poor vegetation.

Since the Paleolithic era, humans have been consumers of game, fish and wild fiber plants, and their evolution has brought about less than 5% change in dietary behavior.

In this book, we review the notion of ecosystem, the history of the human food line from our distant origins to modern man, via the separate branches of the hominids and their current descendants, the great apes. This historical approach to food has enabled us to learn about the foods that have been familiar to us since our origins.

In the section on the geography of food, we describe certain eating habits, to show the extent to which culture influences people's eating habits.

We then went on to observe and detail the diets of certain populations, which show evidence of solid health and longevity.

In conclusion: the modern diet, although largely excessive in proteins, lipids and carbohydrates, is far from providing sufficient quantities of vitamins and minerals. Chemically-grown vegetables, canned foods and other processed foods are very low in nutrients.

These foods are not immune to health problems. In fact, the West suffers from malnutrition and over-nutrition. To compensate for this curious state of affairs, and ensure real health, we need to reduce the quantity of food we eat, and improve its quality.

Our current diet is not adapted to our needs, nor does it take into account our lack of physical activity or our lifestyle habits.

Returning to a prehistoric Paleolithic diet, as some would like to encourage us to do, is not adapted to our current living conditions. Our Paleolithic ancestors ate what nature had to offer: raw, seasonal, unprocessed, natural, unpolluted foods, consumed immediately and without sweeteners like salt and sugar. Foods for which we have had the digestive enzymes for hundreds of thousands of years, and which are therefore easy to digest.

This is where we need to draw inspiration from prehistory, by returning to eating food as it is, without any processing other than that which facilitates digestion. In fact, this is the way of life of the peoples who set us the example today of a healthy diet that enables us to live to a hundred in good health. Everything is available to us, but not everything is useful.

REFERENCES

1. FRATHIA Khalida: *"General Ecology "2nd* year LMD 2023.

2. Claude Faurrie, Christiane Ferra et *&: "Ecologie, approche scientifique et pratique"* 6èEdution 2011.

3. Thierry souccar, *le régime préhistorique, comment l'alimentation des origines peut nous sauver des maladies de civilisation,* indigène édition, 2007.

4. Jean Seignalet, *l'alimentation ou la troisième médecine, coll écologie* humaine, reference work.

5. *Interview with Loren Cordain, professor at the University of Colorado and one of the leaders in prehistoric or Paleolithic nutrition.PNNS*
. http://www. Ianutrition. fr/bien-dans-sa-sante/les-maladies/les-maladies- neurodegeneratives/loren-cordain-le-ble-est-peut-etre-la-pire-des-cereales.html
In an interview with La Nutrition.fr - Thursday, March 31, 2011

6. Theodosius Dobzhansky (1900-1975) *"Nothing in biology makes sense except in the light of evolution."* (1973) "Nothing in biology makes sense except in the light of evolution."

7. Anne Cayot *teQ&mann "The original human diet and naturelle "Memoiie* de find etudes, Institut supérieur de naturopathie (ISUPNAT), Paris 2012.

8. David Reich of Harvard *Medical School in Boston published* in Nature in 2004

9. Nick Patterson, Daniel J. Richter, Sante Gnerre, Eric S. Lander and David Reich, *"Genetic evidence for complex speciation of humans and chimpanzees",* in Nature, vol. 441, no. 7097, June 29, 2006, pp. 1103-1108

1 0.Ogilvie M.D., Curvan B.K. and Trinkaus E. (1989) *"Incidence and*

patterning of dental enamel hypoplasia among the Neandertals", Am. J. Phys. Anthropol. 79: p. 25-41.

1 1.Cépède (M.) and Langellé (M.)> *Economie alimentaire du globe* (Paris, Librairie de Médicis, 1953). De Castro (J.), *Géographie de la faim* (Paris,
Editions ouvrières, 1949). De Castro (J.), Géopolitique de la faim. Economie et humanisme (Paris, Editions ouvrières, 1956). F.A.O., *La situation mondiale de I¹ Alimentation et de I¹ Agriculture* (1953-1954, 1955-1956, Rome).

12. Veyret-Vemer Germaine. *Les différents types de régime alimentaire* : Essai d'interprétation géographique. In: *Revue de géographie alpine,* tome 45, n° 2, 1957. pp. 251-272.

13. *https://books. google, com/books ? id= 6NPMDAAA QBAJ&printsec =frontcover #v=onepage&q&f=false*

14. *https://academic.oup.com/whq/article-abstract/15/4/462/1884227*

15. *https://www.westonaprice.org/the-masai-part-ii-a-glimpse-of-the-masai-diet- at-the-tum-of-the-20th-century-a-land-of-milk-and-honey-bananas-from-afar/*

16. *https://www.ncbi.nlm.nih.gov/pubmed/11507962*

17. *https://muse.jhu.edu/article/578433/summary*

18. *https://www.sciencedirect.com/science/article/pH/088915759290 026G*

19. *https://www.ncbi.nlm.nih.gov/pmc/articles/PMC2638732/*

20. *https://www.ncbi.nlm.nih.gov/pubmed/26567203*

21. *https://www.ncbi.nlm.nih.gov/pmc/articles/PMC5981249/*

22. *https://www. ncbi. nlm. nih.gov/pmc/articles/PMC2367001/*

23. *https://www.nature.com/articles/naturel2820*

24. *https://www.nature.com/articles/nri3430*

25. *https://www. ncbi. nlm. nih.gov/pubmed/22045480*

26. *https://nyaspubs. onlinelibrary.wiley. com/doi/abs/10.1111/j.1
749-
6632.2012.06610.x '*

27. *https://www.ncbi.nlm.nih.gov/pubmed/25051278*
28. *https://healthwyze.org/archive/nutritionandphysicaldegeneration
doctorwesto naprice.pdf*

29. *https://royalsocietypublishing.org/doi/abs/10.1098/rstb.
1991.0115*

30. *https://royalsocietypublishing.org/doi/abs/10.1098/rstb.
1991.0115*

31. *https://www.ncbi.nlm.nih.gov/pubmed/27223304*

32. *https://www.ncbi.nlm.nih.gov/pubmed/27235022*

33. *https://www.ncbi.nlm.nih.gov/pubmed/30050374*

34. *https://www.ncbi.nlm.nih.gov/pubmed/28235195*

35. *https://www.ncbi.nlm.nih.gov/pubmed/27411588*

36. *https://www.ncbi.nlm.nih.gov/pubmed/27411588*

37. *http://stm.sdencemag.org/content/9/377/eaai8700.short*

38. *https://www.ncbi.nlm.nih.gov/pubmed/27239035*

39. *https://www.sciencedirect.com/science/article/pH/S19345909140
01519*

40. *https://www.ncbi.nlm.nih.gov/pmc/articles/PMC5981249/*

41..Doublet F.7à *Poitiers Vegans gain ground* [Internet].
7apoitiers.2015 [cité4févr2017].

Available on: http://www.7apoitiers.fr/enquete/1602/les-vegans-
gagnent 6-u-land.

42.   Van Lennepkade N. *Vegetarianism in Europe and the world*
(map) [Intemet].Vegactu. [cited4feb2017].

Available at: http://www.vegactu.com/actualite/carte -des-vegetariens-
dans-le-monde-6921/

43.   EVANA *Vegetarians around the worlden* [Internet], 2013 [cited
4 Feb 2017]. Available from:

http : //www.evana. org/index.php ?id=70650

44.   Lamisse F. *The vegetarian diet.* Médecine Mal Métaboliques,
March 2013;7(2):109àll3.

45.   Dupont F, Reus E. *Who are the new vegetarians?* - Sociology and
vegetarianism. 3 Janvier2012. (35).

46.   Beeson L. *The adventist health advantage--Dialogue.* Dialogue
Univ. 1999;11(2):8-11.

47.   Lecerf J-M. Particularités du sénior végétarien, sept
2009;3(4):380 à 385.

48.   *A balanced diet* - AVF [Internet], [cited 12 June 2016]. Available
from: http://www.vegetarisme.fr/comment-devenir-
vegetarien/alimentation- equilibree/

49.   Ministèie du travail, de l'emploi et de la santé. *Programme*

national nutrition santé 2011 -2015. 2011.

50. Duhamel J-F, Brouard J. L'eau et l'hydratation : *une nécessité pour la vie.* mars2010;23: 9-12.

51. *Shewry PR, Hey SJ. The contribution of wheat to human diet and health.* FoodEnergy Secur. Oct 2015;4(3):178-202.

52. Eschwege E, Charles M-A, Basevant A, Moisan C, Bonnélye G, Touboul C, et al. *National epidemiological survey on overweight and obesity* 2012. .

53. Clarys P, Deriemaeker P, Huybrechts M, Mullie P. *Dietary pattern analysis: a comparison between matched vegetarian and omnivorous subjects.* Nutr J. June 2013; 12(82): 1-6.

54. Guenther PM, Kirkpatrick SI, Reedy J, Krebs-Smith SM, Buckman DW, Dodd KW, et al. *The healthy Eating Indes-2010 Is a valid and reliable measure of diet quad ty according to the 2010 dietary guidelines for americans.* J Nutr. 22 Jan2014; 1-9.

55. Key TJ, Davey GK, Appleby PN. *Health benefits of a vegetarian diet. Proc Nutr* Soc. May 1999;58(2):271-5.

56. Fraser GE. *Vegetarian diets: -what do we know of thei r effects on common chronic diseases?*Am J ClinNutr. 2009;89(Supplement): 1607S-1612S.

57. Pineau J, Kapitaniak B. *Determination of theoretical weight in 20-year-old French patients: relationship between underweight or overweight and body mass index* (BMI). 2004. (8):93-100.

58. Bouillanne O, Morineau G, Dupont C, Coulombel I, Vincent J -P, Nicolis I, et al. *Geriatric Nutritional Risk Index: a new index for*

evaluating at-risk elderly medical patients. AmJ ClinNutr. 1 Oct 2005;82(4):777-83.

59. Bardin C. *Evaluation of different weight descriptors in the obese subject using a population pharmacokinetic model - application to metformin, morphine and imatinib -.* Paris Descartes; 2012.

60.WHO I *Diabetes* [Internet], WHO. [cited 2016 Nov 5]. Available from:

http: //www.who. int/me diacentre/factsheets/fs312/en/

61. Key TJ, Appleby PN, Rosell MS. *Health effects of vegetarian and vegan diets.* ProcNutr Soc. Feb 2006;65(l):35-41.

62. Key TJ, Fraser GE, Thorogood M, Appleby PN, Beral V, Reeves G, et al. *Mortality in vegetarians and nonvegetarians: detailed findings from a collaborative analysis of 5 prospective studies.* Am J Clin Nutr. 1999;70(Supplement):516S-524S.

63. Battaglia Richi E, Baumer B, Conrad B, Darioli R, Schmid A, Keller U. *Health aspects of meat consumption.* Forum Med Suisse. 2015; 15(24):566-72.

64. Huang T, Yang B, Zheng J, Li G, Wahlqvist ML, Li D. *Cardiovascular disease mortality and cancer incidence in vegetarians: a meta-analysis and* systematic review. Ann Nutr Metab. June 1, 2012;(60):233-40.

65. Debiase SG, Fernandes SFC, Gianini RJ, Duarte JLG. *Vegetarian diet and cholesterol and triglycerides levels.* ArqBras Cardiol. 2007;88(l):32-6.

66. Wang F, Zheng J, Yang B, Jiang J, Fu Y, Li D. *Effects OfVegetarian Diets on Blood Lipids: A Systematic Review and Meta-Analysis of Randomized Controlled Trials.* J Am Heart Assoc

Cardiovasc Cerebrovasc Dis. 27 Oct 2015;4(10).

67. Chang-Gaude J, Hermann S, Eilber U, SteindorfKaren. Lifestyle *Determinants and Mortality in German Vegetarians and Health-Conscious Persons: Results of a 21-yearFollow-up.* CancerEpidemiol Biomarkers Prev. April 2005;14(4):963-8.

68. Segasothy M, Phillips PA. *Vegetarian diet: panacea for modem lifestyle diseases?* Q J Med. 1999;92:531-44.

69. Pilis W, Stec K, Zych M, Pilis A. *Health benefits and risk associated with adopting a vegetarian diet.* Rocz Panstw Zakl Hig. 2014;65(l):9-14.

70. Thériault S, Giguère Y, Douville P. *Elevated creatininemia.* Médecin Qué. Dec 2014;49(12).

71. Barsotti G, Cupisti A, Morelli E, Ciardella F, Giovannetti S. *Vegan supplement diet in nephrotic syndrome.* Nephrol Dial Transplant. 1990;5(suppl l):75-7.
72. Lin C-K, Lin D-J, Yen C-H, Chen S-C, Chen C-C, Wang T-Y, et al. *Comparison of Renal Function and Other Health Outcomes in Vegetarians versus Omnivores in Taiwan.* JHealthPopul Nutr. Oct 2010;28(5):470-5.

73. Tantamango-Bartley Y, Jaceldo-Siegl K, Fan J, Fraser G. *Vegetarian Diets and the Incidence of Cancer in a Low-risk Population.* Cancer Epidemiol Biomarkers Prev. 1 Feb 2013;22(2):286-94.41.

74. Giovannucci E, Rimm EB, Stampfer MJ, Colditz GA, Ascherio A, Willett WC. *Intake of fat, meat, and fiber in relation to risk of colon cancer in men.* CancerRes. Imai 1994;54: 2390-7.

75. Fraser GE. *Association between diet and cancer, ischemic heart disease, and all -cause mortality in non-Hispanic white California Seventh-day Adventists.* Am J ClinNutr. 1999;70(Supplement):532S-538S.

76. Salehi M, Moradi-Lakeh M, Salehi MH, Nojomi M, Kolahdooz F. *Meat, fish, and esophageal cancer risk: a systematic review and dose-response metaanalysis.* Nutr Rev.2013;71(5):257-67.

77. *Larousse E. Encyclopédie Larousse en ligne - maladies transmises par l'eau et les* a//'me "tó[Intemet].[cited 13 Dec 2016].Disponible sur: http : //www.larousse. fr/encycl opedie/medi cal/mal adies_transmise s_par_le au_et
   food s/185308

TS. Camart-perie A. *Salmonella, bovine salmonellosis, state of the art, epidemiology in France.* [France]: Ecole vétérinaire de Maisons-Alfort; 2006.

79.*Salmonellosis* [Internet], Institut Pasteur. 2013 [cited 13 Dec 2016]. Available from: https://www.pasteur.fr/fr/institut-pasteur/presse/fichesinfo/salmonellose
80. *Hepatitis* A *transmission* [Hepatites Info Service] [Internet], Hepatites Info Service.org. 2013 [cited 15 Dec 2016]. Available from: https://www.hepatites -info-service.org/?Hepatite-A- Transmission

81. *Aide-memoire / Hepatitis A / Viral hepatitis / Infectious diseases / Thematic files/ Home [Internet]. Institut de veille sanitaire,* [cited 22 Dec 2016] .Available from: http://invs.santepubliquefrance. fr/Dossiersthematiques/Mal adies-infectieuses/Hepatites-virales/Hepatite-A/Aide-memoire

& !.*Parasitoses digestives : Iambliase, taeniasis, ascariasis, oxyurosis, amoebiasis, hydatidosis* [Internet], 2004 Avri 1 [cited 29

Dec 2016]; Faculté de médecine de
Grenoble.Disponiblesur:http://www.sante.ujfgrenoble.fr/sante/corpus/
disciplines/p arasitomyco/parasito/100/leconimprim. pdf

83. Vaillant V, De Valk H, Baron E. *Morbidity and mortality due to foodborne infectious diseases in France* [Internet], Institut de veille sanitaire;2004.Disponiblesur:
http://opac.invs.sante.fr/doc_num.php?explnum_id=5780

84. *Bouteille* B. *Epidemiology of cysticercosis and neurocysticercosis.* Médecine Santé Trop. June 1, 2014;(24):367-74.

85. WHO I *TaeniasisZcysti cercóse* [Internet], WHO. april 16 [cited 29 Dec 2016]. Available from: http://www.who. int/mediacentre/factsheets/fs376/en/

86. Ramage-Morin PL. *Creuztfeldt-Jakob disease.* StatCan. July 2004;15(4):51-4.

87. Roels S, De Meyer G, *Vanopdenbosch E. Bovine spongiform encephalopathy and variant Creutzfeldt Jakob disease: some information concerning origin, diagnosis, epidemiology, risk analysis and future.* AnnMéd Vét. 2001;(145):333-41.
88. Capek I. *Suspicions of Creutzfeldt Jakob disease and other human transmissible spongiform encephalopathies in 1996 and 1997.* BEH. August 24, 1999;(34).

89. Coulthart MB, Cashman NR Variant Creutzfeldt Jakob disease: *a summary of current scientific knowledge in relation to public health.* Can Med Assoc Its Licens. IOjuill 2001;165(l):51-8.

90. Weissenberger S, Sampaio daSilva D, Schetagne R. *The ecosystem approach to population health: the case of mercury exposure in*

riparian communities in the Amazon and northern Quebec. Dév Durable Territ. 2013;4(2):1-28.

91. De morais SS. *Neurotoxic effects of mercury exposure in the Brazilian Amazon* [Internet], 2006 [cited 14 Jan 2017]. Available from: http://www.archipel. uqam. ca/3203/ 1/M9484. pdf

92. Briand P, Demoncheaux J-P, Mazenot C. *Environmental pollution by mercury in French Guiana.* Synthèse bibliographique. Médecine Armées, February 2007;35(l):51-6.

93. *Mercury (chemistry).* In: Wikipedia [Internet], 2017 [cited 14 Jan 2017]. Di sponible sur:

https://fr.wikipediaorg/w/index.php?title=Mercure_(chemistry)&oldid =133560684

94. Craig WJ. *Iron status of vegetarians.* Am J Clin Nutr. May 1, 1994; 59(5):1233S-1237S.

95.   Leonard AJ, Chalmers KA, Collins CE, Patterson AJ. *The effect of nutrition knowledge and dietary iron intake on iron status in young women.* 2014;(81):225-31.
96. Hunt JR. *Bioavailability of iron, zinc, and other trace minerals from vegetarian diets.* AmJ ClinNutr. 1 Sep 2003;78(3):633S-639S.

97. Hurrell R, *Egli I. Iron bioavailability and dietary reference values.* Am J Clin Nutr. 2010;91S:1461S-1467S.

98. Chalon S. *Polyunsaturated fatty acids and cognitive function.* OCL journal. July-August 2001;8(4):317-20.

99. Guesnet P, Alessandri J-M, Astorg P, Pifferi F, Lavialle M. *The major physiological roles played by polyunsaturated fatty acids (PUFAs).* OCL journal, sept 2005;12(5-6):333-43.

100. Bourre J-M. *Dietary omega-3 fatty acids and neuropsychiatry.* OCL journal. 5janv 2015;1 l(4):362-70.

I OLDumas C, Kalonji E, Thomann C, Gnanou J. *Omega-3 fatty acids and the cardiovascular system: nutritional interest and claims.* In AFSSA éditeur; 2003 [cited 2016 May 7]. Available from: https: //www. anses.fr/en/system/files/NUT-Ra-omega3. pdf

102. Girardet JP. *Nutritional benefits and potential risks of fish consumption.* Réal Pédiatriques, Sept 2012;(172).

103. Dubois V, Breton S, Linder M, Fanni J, Parmentier M. *Proposed classification of vegetable sources of fatty acids according to their nutritional profile.* OCLjoumal. Jan 2008;15(l):56-75.

104. Uddin MK, Juraimi AS, Hossain MS, Nahar MAU, Ali ME, Rahman MM. *Purslane Weed (Portulaca olerácea): A Prospective Plant Source of Nutrition, Omega-3 Fatty Acid, and Antioxidant Attributes.* Sci World J. Feb 10, 2014; 2014.
105. Serraj K, Federici L, Ciobanu E, Andnes E. *Vitamin deficiencies: from symptom to treatment,* mt. nov 2007;13(6):411-20.

106. Elmadfa I, Singer I. *Vitamin B-12 and homocysteine status among vegetarians: a global perspective.* AmJ ClinNutr. 2009;89(suppl):1693-8.

107. Benhamou C-L, Souberbielle J-C, Cortet B, Fardellone P, Gauvain J-B, Thomas T. *Vitamin D in adults: recommendations of the GRIO.* Presse Médicale, July-August 2011;40(7-8):673-82.

108. Dawson-Hughes B, Heaney RP, Holick MF, Lips P, Meunier PJ, Vieth R. *Estimates of optimal vitamin D status.* Int Osteoporos Found Natl Osteoporos Found. March 18, 2005; 16:713-6.

109. Cahn G. *Vitamin D: from biology to practice.* Ann Gérontologie. Sept 2009;(special):4-16.

110. Tripkovic L, Lambert H, Hart K, Smith CP, Bucca G, Penson S, et al. *Comparison of vitamin D2 and vitamin D3 supplementation in raising serum 25-hydroxyvitamin D status: a systematic review and mete-analysis.* Am J Clin Nutr. 2012;95:1357-64.

111. Vemay M, Sponga M, Salanave B, Oléko A, Deschamps V, Malon A, et al. *Vitamin D status of the adult population in France: l'étude nationale nutrition santé* (ENNS, 2006-2007). Bull Épidémiologique Hebd. 24 Apr 2012;(16-17):189-94.

112. *Calcium* | Anses - Agence nationale de sécurité sanitaire de France
l'alimentation, de l'environnement et du travail [Internet], 2016 [cited5feb2017].Available from: https://www.anses.fr/fr/content/le-calcium.

113. Mangels AR. Bone nutrients for vegetarians.Am J Clin Nutr.2014;100(Suppl.):469-75.
114. Tucker KL. Vegetarian diets and bones status. Am J Clin Nutr. 2014; 100(Suppl.):329-35.

115. Wang Y-F, Chiu J-S, Chuang M-H, Chiu J-E, Lin C-L. *Bone mineral density of vegetarian and non- vegetarian adults in Tarwan.* Asia Pac J Clin Nutri. 2008;17(l):101-6.

116. Ayoubi J-M, Hirt R, Badiou W, Hininger-Favier I, Favier M,

Zraik- Ayoubi F, et al. *Nutrition et femme enceinte*. Elsevier Masson SAS Paris. 2012;l-13.

117. Finley DA, Lonnerdal B, Dewey KG, Grivetti LE. *Breast milk composition: fat content and fatty acid composition in vegetarians and non-vegetarians*. Am J ClinNutr. 1 Apr 1985;41(4):787-800.

118. Amit M. *Vegetarian diets in children and adolescents*. Paediatr Child Health. 2010;15(5):309-14.

119. Anses *points to risks associated with feeding infants drinks other than breast milk and substitutes\ Anses - Agence nationale de sécurité sanitaire de l'alimentation, de l'environnement et du travail* [Internet], [cited15janv2017].Disponiblesur: https://www.anses.fr/fr/content/l%E2%80%99anses-pointe-les-risques- li%C3%A9s-%C3%A0- l%E2%80%99feeding-infants-with-other-beverages-0

120. Jacobs C, Dwyer JT. *Vegetarian children: appropriate and inappropriate diets*. AmJClinNutr. 1 Sep 1988;48(3):811-8.

121.Specker BL, Black A, Alien L, Morrow F. Vitamin B-12: *low milk concentrations are related to low serum concentrations in vegetarian w omen and to methylmalonic aciduria in their infants*. Am J Clin Nutr. 1 Dec 1990; 52(6):1073-6.
122. Foster M, Chu A, Petocz P, Samman S. *Effect of vegetarian diets on zinc status: a systematic review and meta-analysis of studies in humans*. Soc Chem Ind. 2013;(93):2362-71.

123 Sanders TA, Reddy S. *Vegetarian diets and children. Am J CHn Nutr*. May 1, 1994;59(5):1176S-1181S.

124. Campbell WW, Barton ML, Cyr-Campbell D, Davey SL,

Beard JL, Parise G, et al. *Effects of an omnivorous diet compared with an Iactoovovegetarian diet on resistance-training-induced changes in body composition and skeletal muscle in older men.* Am J Clin Nutr. Dec 1, 1999;70(6):1032-9.

125. Allepaerts S, Delcourt S, Petermans J. *Les troubles de la déglutition du sujet âgé : un problème trop souvent sous estimé.* Rev Med Liège. 2008; 63(12):715-21.

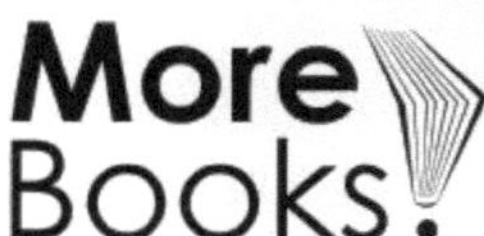

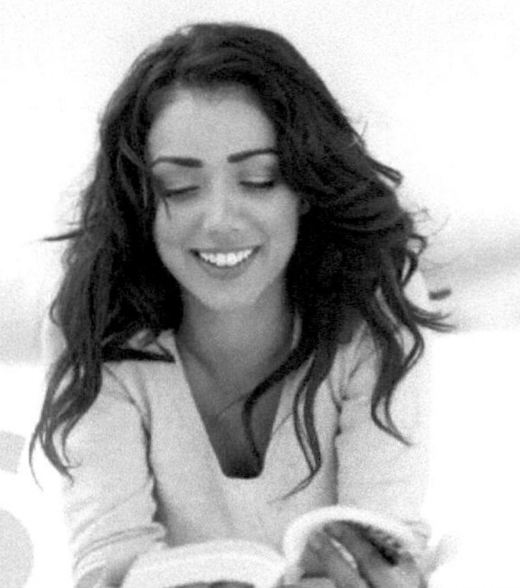

I want morebooks!

Buy your books fast and straightforward online - at one of world's fastest growing online book stores! Environmentally sound due to Print-on-Demand technologies.

Buy your books online at
www.morebooks.shop

Kaufen Sie Ihre Bücher schnell und unkompliziert online – auf einer der am schnellsten wachsenden Buchhandelsplattformen weltweit! Dank Print-On-Demand umwelt- und ressourcenschonend produzi ert.

Bücher schneller online kaufen
www.morebooks.shop

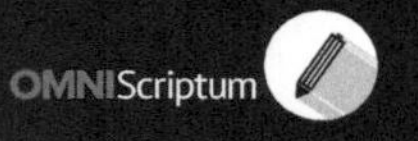

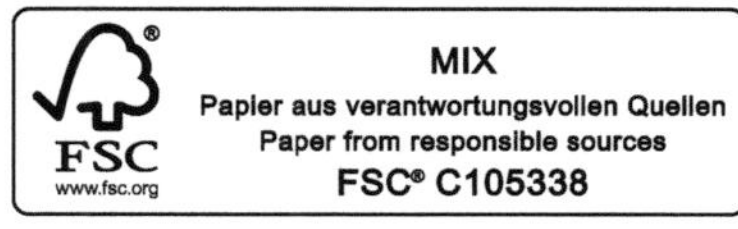

Printed by Books on Demand GmbH, Norderstedt / Germany